HEALTH AND HAPPINESS:
SIMPLE, SAFE AND SOUND SYSTEMS AND SOLUTIONS

Emanuel Cheraskin, M.D., D.M.D.

Bio-Communications Press
3100 North Hillside Avenue
Wichita, Kansas 67219

Copyright © 1989
This book may not be reproduced in whole or in part, by mimeograph or any other means, without permission.
For information address:

BIO-COMMUNICATIONS PRESS
3100 North Hillside Avenue
Wichita, Kansas 67219 USA

ISBN 0-942333-05-5
Library of Congress Catalog Card Number: 88-62803

First Edition

Published in the United States of America

The information contained in this book has been compiled from a variety of sources and is subject to differences of opinion and interpretation. This book is not intended as a source of medical advice, and any questions, general or specific, should be addressed to the reader's nutrition-oriented physician.

BCP and Bio-Communications Press are service marks of The Olive W. Garvey Center for the Improvement of Human Functioning, Inc.

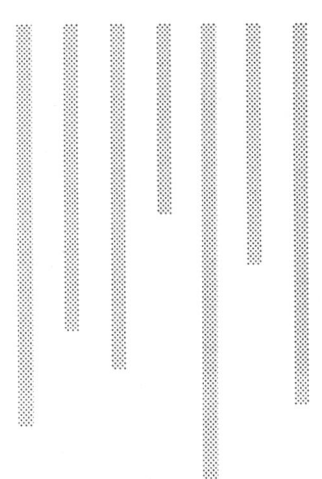

TABLE OF CONTENTS

Kudos	v
In the beginning...then and now	vii
The gist of the story	ix
Part A: The Prologue	1
1. Who's in Charge (of Your Body)?	3
Part B: Problems	17
2. Are You as Bushed (as Most People Think They Are)?	19

3.	Are You Going to Get Cancer?	41
4.	How's Your Arthritis?	57
5.	Are You (Literally) Dying to be Thin?	73
6.	How's Your (Good and Bad) Cholesterol?	89
7.	Low Blood Sugar—the Nondisease!	109
8.	Don't Let Stress Kill You!	127
9.	What's Your "Financial" State of Health?	151
10.	How's Your Workplace Health?	169
11.	Other Problems	187
12.	Finally...Are You a Happy Person?	209

Part C: Solutions	223
13. How Fantastic Are You?	225
14. How Well do You Eat?	247
15. Why Do You "Really" Smoke?	271
16. Are You Drinking Too Much (Alcohol)?	293
17. How Active Are You?	313
18. Sleep: The Other Third of Your Life	331
19. Other Solutions	349

Part D: The Epilogue	371
20. Are You 40 Going on 70.. Or 70 Going on 40?	373

The Index	395

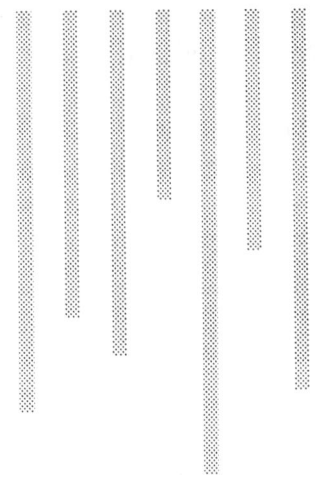

KUDOS

There's no question but that writing a book is a big job! Compassionate and creative colleagues are essential.

And I have been fortunate in that regard.

I want to thank my secretary/co-worker Sara Gay who was responsible for the reading and collation of literally thousands of pages of text and references. Obviously, **HEALTH AND HAPPINESS** would not have been possible without it. I want to take this time to recognize the Wichita people, namely Barbara Nichols of Bio-Communications Press who took these thousands of pages and helped arrange them in meaningful fashion and Lisa Hostetler who designed the cover.

This book is obviously based upon a series of self-administrable and self-scorable questionnaires. You will find that we have acknowledged throughout this text the scores of investigators for their fundamental research resulting in many practical quizes.

Finally, **HEALTH AND HAPPINESS** could not have come to pass without the effort and extraordinary insight of Hugh D. Riordan, M.D., President of The Olive W. Garvey Center and Bio-Communications Press.

One more important addendum. Titling a book can and is often a painful and prolonged process. Not so for **HEALTH AND HAPPINESS**. The label seemed right then in 1984. It seems right now! During our final bibliographic check, we chanced across a fascinating book by Doctor H. H. Bloomfield and R. B. Kory entitled "The Holistic Way to Health and Happiness: A New Approach to Complete Lifetime Wellness" published in 1978. While the titles bear some semblance; the books are vastly different. Notwithstanding, they have not only made a contribution to the reading public but have also significantly advanced our thinking.

We look forward to your constructive criticisms so that hopefully **HEALTH AND HAPPINESS** can continue to grow and mature into a truly successful self-help instrument.

E. Cheraskin, M.D., D.M.D.

IN THE BEGINNING
... THEN AND NOW

In the beginning...and looking back over these many years, I believe my medical training may be summarized as a series of exercises. These experiences were intended by means of varied and diverse tools designed to help people by supplying them with a **specific** diagnosis and then to provide them with a **specific** solution. I was impressed **then**, and continue to be **now**, with the fact that a patient suffering excruciating pain, for example because of a broken leg, could literally walk out of the office in unbelievable comfort minutes after receiving a pain killer and having a cast applied. I was **then** and **now** just as overwhelmed that a glob of gold can be centrifused and then fitted in microns to fill a tooth.

Then...

After graduation I came to learn that these magnificent tools were, almost without exception, **mechanical** devices intended to resolve **mechanical** problems. Out there in the real world I also discovered that most so-called medical problems were biologic, not mechanical and the armamentaria at my disposal were largely ineffective. What troubled me more than anything else though was recognizing how powerless I was to help people with most of their ailments. It came to be almost like a vision. The majority of physical complaints constituted for-want-of-a-better-phrase a **nonspecific** syndrome of sickness and resulted from the **nonspecific** breaking of the rules of sensible lifestyle. This obviously can only be rectified by the patient.

And now...

I know that **self**-help begins with **self**-recognition of the problem.

THE GIST OF THE STORY

The universality of **health and happiness** can be demonstrable in different peoples irrespective of age, sex, color and creed. It almost seems as if there is no rhyme or reason to **health and happiness**. But there is...and it's lifestyle. Those who seem to be well are characterized by positive social habits (pluses). The unhealthy and unhappy are laden with poor lifestyle (minuses). Would you believe...it's just that simple!

THE PROLOGUE

People are surely different...some are big and others are small...there are the fat and the thin...and the mad and the glad. All of us, by act if not by word, have some conscious or otherwise notion of why we're well and what happens to make us sick. In the final analysis, there are two extremes of people's belief systems regarding the causes of **health and happiness**. At one pole there are folks who hold to the idea that they have absolutely no control over their own physical and mental well-being; at the other limit are those who fervently believe that they are totally in command.

Clearly, those in the former group need not continue reading this monograph since there's nothing they can do to modify their own **health and happiness**. Fortunately, most of us aren't at the extremes. Generally, we would agree that we're in part (and we'll try to find out how much) responsible for our health/disease state. Consequently, other than the very far-out earthling, this book can serve well for most people.

Where to begin?

Why not start with a questionnaire that will provide us with some measurable inkling of our **health and happiness**.

1

WHO'S IN CHARGE (OF YOUR BODY)?

Who's **really** responsible for your health? Well, there are scores of opinions and bunches of rationalizations depending upon who one asks.

In the summer of 1964, Norman Cousins, the distinguished former editor of the Saturday Review, was diagnosed as having ankylosing spondylitis, a devastating disease that eventually disintegrates the connective tissue of the spine. When his doctor issued the grim verdict that he only had "one chance in five hundred" of recovering, Cousins decided it was about time to take an active interest in his own case.

"All this gave me a great deal to think about," he recalled in his book **Anatomy of an Illness**. "Up to that time I had been more or less disposed to let the doctors worry about my condition. But now I felt a compulsion to get into the act. It seemed clear to me that if I was to be that one in five hundred I had better be something more than a passive observer."

Cousins goes on to outline in great detail how he developed his own treatment regime, formed a partnership with his physician, and ultimately broke free from the clutches of this crippling, degenerative disease.

Cousins demonstrated by his action the two limits with regard to "who's in charge (of your body)?". On the one hand, many people believe that illness is determined by uncontrollable outside forces, like God, IBM, doctors, or whoever runs this world (depending upon your religious persuasion). These folk have it in their heads that they have no control over illness, that sickness is brought on by outside forces and their hands are figuratively tied when it comes to change. At the other end of the spectrum are those who believe that breaking nature's laws invites ill-health. These people passionately perceive that modifiable lifestyle ingredients, like the consumption of alcohol, coffee or tea, tobacco, physical activity and diet, play a significant part in good health maintenance. They feel strongly that their own actions exert a primary influence on their health/sickness status. In the real world, most of us hold an opinion somewhere in between these two limiting poles.

Laced through this chapter you'll frequently encounter a scientific term called **health locus of control**. It's a testing designation which allows a grading of the extent of control over your health destiny. The validity has been well substantiated in more than 2,000 studies over the past two decades. For example, there's a reasonably accurate test already available which provides significant prediction regarding the success of orthodontic treatment (p. 11). Additionally, one can anticipate prevention mindedness in oral health (p. 13).

Identifying who you really believe is in charge of your body is an important and critical first step to getting the most out of the questionnaires in subsequent chapters. After all, if you don't know where you are, how can you possibly tell where you're going?

In what follows, each item is a belief statement with which you may or may not agree. For every item insert the number that represents the extent to which you disagree or agree. The more strongly you concur, the higher the number will be. The more fervently you disagree with the statement, the lower the number. Make absolutely sure that you answer every item and mark only one number. This is a measure of your personal beliefs; obviously, there are no right or wrong answers.

Please answer these questions carefully, but don't spend too much time on any one. Try to respond to each point independently. When making a choice, avoid being influenced by your earlier decisions. It's important that you answer according to your own beliefs, not by how you should believe or how you think we want you to believe. Simply be truthful.

Please note the scoring system:
1 = strongly disagree
2 = moderately disagree
3 = lightly disagree
4 = lightly agree
5 = moderately agree
6 = strongly agree

1. If I get sick, it is my own behavior, that determines how soon I get well again.

2. I am in control of my health.

3. When I get sick, I am to blame.

4. The main thing that affects my health is what I myself do.

5. If I take care of myself, I can avoid illness.

6. If I take the right actions, I can stay healthy.

7. If I become sick, I have the power to make myself well again.

8. I am directly responsible for my health.

9. Whatever goes wrong with my health is my own fault.

10. My physical well-being depends on how well I take care of myself.

11. When I feel ill, I know it is because I have not been taking care of myself properly.

12. I can pretty much stay healthy by taking good care of myself.

13. No matter what I do, if I am going to get sick, I will get sick.

14. Most things that affect my health happen to me by accident.

15. Luck plays a big part in determining how soon I will recover from an illness.

16. My good health is largely a matter of good fortune.

17. No matter what I do, I'm likely to get sick.

18. If it's meant to be, I will stay healthy.

19. Often I feel that no matter what I do, if I am going to get sick, I will get sick.

20. It seems that my health is greatly influenced by accidental happenings.

21. When I am sick, I just have to let nature run its course.

22. When I stay healthy, I'm just plain lucky.

23. Even when I take care of myself, it's easy to get sick.

24. When I become ill, it's a matter of fate.

25. Having regular contact with my physician is the best way for me to avoid illness.

26. Whenever I don't feel well, I should consult a medically trained professional.

27. My family has a lot to do with my becoming sick or staying healthy.

28. Health professionals control my health.

29. When I recover from an illness, it's usually because other people (for example, doctors, nurses, family, friends) have been taking good care of me.

30. Regarding my health, I can only do what my doctor tells me to do.

31. If I see an excellent doctor regularly, I am less likely to have health problems.

32. I can only maintain my health by consulting health professionals.

33. Other people play a big part in whether I stay healthy or become sick.

34. Health professionals keep me healthy.

35. The type of care I receive from other people is what is responsible for how well I recover from an illness.

36. Following doctor's orders to the letter is the best way for me to stay healthy.

Here's how to score this questionnaire. First, add your responses to questions 1 through 12 and put the total in the box just below:

☐ **Internal Health Locus of Control (IHLC)**

The minimum possible score is 12 and the maximum is 72. It's rare indeed to score at either end. The average is 50.4, suggesting, at least to some extent, that we're personally responsible for our well-being. These questions and the score derived from them constitute what is referred to as the **Internal Health Locus of Control (IHLC)**. The bigger the number, the more you're in charge! A practical consequence is included (p. 12). A study has been done of children of intact versus divorced families showing significantly higher internality of children and especially boys of separated family units.

Now total up the scores for questions 13 through 24. Collectively, they constitute the **Chance Health Locus of Control (CHLC)**. Put the score in the box below.

☐ **Chance Health Locus of Control (CHLC)**

One may conclude that the higher the score, the more you believe in pure chance. The range is from a low of 12 to a high of 72. It's highly unlikely that you'll find yourself at either extreme. The average for the **CHLC** is 31.0, which indicates most of us do not believe very strongly that chance is a serious factor in determining our health. For those interested in more information about your **gutsy index**, there's a very informative questionnaire which appeared in the January 1988 issue of Prevention Magazine developed by Ralph Keys. For more particulars regarding his concepts, see resources (p. 13).

Finally, total up the responses to questions 25 through 36. Again, the range is from a low of 12 to a high of 72 with an average of 40.9. Now insert your total score in the box below.

☐ **Powers Health Locus of Control (PHLC)**

These questions are aimed at determining how much control you think others, like God or doctors, have in dominating your health. This section is known as **Powers Health Locus of Control (PHLC)**. The higher the score, the more you believe powerful others have total control over your health. Interestingly enough, these numbers suggest that just about equal percentages of the population are willing or not to attribute their problems to outside influences.

The three combined tests you've just completed are subsets of the **Multidimensional Health Locus of Control (MHLC)**, an instrument developed by Kenneth A. Wallston of Vanderbilt University and Barbara Strudler Wallston at George Peabody College. We wish to take this opportunity to thank these researchers for granting us permission to cite this extraordinary piece of work. Incidentally, Doctors Wallston and Wallston have provided other relevant published material which is referred to in Resources at the end of this chapter.

How you respond to the rest of the questionnaires in this book will clearly be a function of how **internal** or **external** you are or wish to be.

As you proceed, you'll discover we've provided additional resources at the end of each chapter to help guide those of you who desire to find out more about a particular questionnaire, its meaning, and when applicable, where to go for help or guidance.

RESOURCES

1. Duke, M. P. and Cohen, B.
   Locus of Control as an Indicator of Patient Cooperation: Implications for Preventive Dentistry.
   Journal of the American College of Dentists 42: #3, 174-178, July 1975.

   The combined efforts of an associate professor of psychology at Emory University in Atlanta, and a practicing dentist demonstrate the relationship of locus of control in the maintenance of oral hygiene in an orthodontic practice. Using a combination of tests, the authors show how one can predict which children are going to be good patients and which ones are going to be difficult in a private orthodontic practice.

2. Jordan-March, M. and Neutra, R.

Relationship of Health Locus of Control to Lifestyle Change Programs
Research in Nursing and Health 8: #1, 3-11, March, 1985.

These researchers examined the attitudes and physical makeup of 339 people who participated in a lifestyle change program. Weight, blood pressure, low density lipoproteins, triglycerides and cholesterol were checked at the beginning of the study, after 24 days in a residential program, and again six months later. From admission to discharge there were significant changes in scores that reflected how these people perceived **who's in charge**.

3. Kalter, N., Alpern, D., Spence, R. and Plunkett, J. W.
Locus of Control in Children of Divorce
Journal of Personality Assessment 48: #3, 410-414, August 1984.

Locus of control scores, or attitudes, were compared for third and fifth grade boys and girls from intact versus families where the parents are divorced. The results suggest that fifth graders more than third graders, boys more than girls, and those with divorced parents more than the intact group, exhibited higher internality in their locus of control scores. These observations strongly suggest that a divorce in the family during childhood bears a significant influence on how much personal control these children feel they have over their own lives.

4. Kent, G. G., Matthews, R. M., and White, F.H.
Locus of Control and Oral Health
Journal of the American Dental Association 109: #1, 67-69, July 1984.

A behavioral scientist joins forces with two dentists in England to study factors which contribute to success in preventive dentistry. Using a simple, self-administered questionnaire, they concluded that patients whose oral health was rated as good scored in a more internal fashion. Those patients whose oral health was scored as moderate or poor showed a low internal grade, suggesting that locus of control beliefs are important in the design of preventative programs on a personalized basis.

5. Keys, R.
Chancing it: Why we Take Risks
1985. Boston, Little Brown and Company

Ralph Keys, in this fascinating book, confronts the issue of why we so often take chances as it takes a provocative, indepth look into the psychologic and physiologic thirst we all have whether we indulge in it or not. As he sees it, a risk is not derived from an actuarial table, but from our own innermost, subjective feelings; it's "any act one is afraid of taking." The author concludes that taking risks is a necessary and healthy thing to do, but "the American way of risk" has traditionally glorified physical daring at the expense of other kinds, and has created vicarious forms of risk behavior that leave us hungry for the real thing. Instead, he offers us some perceptive guidance in seeking for ourselves what he calls genuine risks, those based less on danger than on the authenticity of our unique, individual feelings.

6. Schlenk, E. A. and Hart, L. K.
Relationship Between Health Locus of Control, Health Value, and Social Support and Compliance of Persons with Diabetes Mellitus
Diabetes Care 7 :#6, 566-574, November/December 1984.

Thirty diabetics were interviewed with questionnaires that measured independent variables of health locus of control, health value, and perceived social support. Self-reporting and direct observations were used to measure the dependent variable, compliance with insulin administration, diet, exercise, the management of low blood sugar, self-monitoring of blood glucose and foot care prescriptions. A statistically significant relationship was found between a number of variables, including health locus of control.

7. Strickland, B. R.
Internal-External Expectancies and Health-Related Behaviors
Journal of Consulting and Clinical Psychology 46: #6, 1192-1211, December 1978.

This review from the Department of Psychology at the University of Massachusetts outlines the research on internal-external (I-E) locus of control expectancies, along with health attitudes and behaviors. Included is a detailed analysis of the theoretical background of the I-E construct. Particular attention is assigned to I-E in relation to health knowledge, precautionary health practices, responses to physical disorders, psychologic responding, psychologic disturbances, and responses to psychologic therapy.

8. Wallston, K. A., Maides, S. and Wallston, B. S.
Health-Related Information Seeking as a Function of Health-Related Locus of Control and Health Value
Journal of Research in Personality 10: #2, 215-222, June 1976.

Two experiments are described which test the theory that seeking information about health is a combined function of an individual's locus of control beliefs and how much value that person assigns to health in general. Utilizing a health-related measure of locus of control, internal subjects who valued health highly chose more pamphlets about their particular health condition, in this case hypertension, than did internal—low health value subjects or externals.

9. Wallston, B. S. and Wallston, K. A.
Locus of Control and Health: A Review of the Literature
Health Education Monographs 6: #1, 107-117,

Spring 1978.

Locus of control or who a person believes is in charge of his or her health, has shown some promise in predicting and explaining specific health-related behaviors. This research reviews the utility of the locus of control in an attempt to understand smoking reduction, birth control utilization, weight loss, information-seeking, adherence to medication regimens, and other health behaviors.

10. Wallston, K. A. and Wallston, B. S.
Who is Responsible for Your Health? The Construct of Health Locus of Control
In Sanders, G. and Suls, J.
Social Psychology of Health and Illness.
1982, Hillsdale, New Jersey, Lawrence Erlbaum & Associates, pp. 65-95.

This thirty page review examines the overall issue. There are sections devoted to the theoretical framework, the available health locus of control scales and the followup of responses to health care interventions. A detailed bibliographic section is included.

B

THE PROBLEMS

What do we mean when we say, "I have a **problem.**?" In some instances, what we're really communicating is the presence of an unsolved symptom (parenthetic mention should be made that, by general agreement, this is a subjective observation reported by an individual and usually incapable of being measured). Who hasn't heard, "Everything's fine except that I have a headache." In other cases, the **problem** consists of a sign (this is conceded to be an objective finding which can be corroborated). "I'm perfectly well except for high blood pressure."

To many, symptoms and signs per se are often not viewed as revealing. "I'm fine. All I need to do is lose a few pounds." But there's no monopoly of definitions. A biochemical aberration can just as readily signify a **problem**. "They tell me the only thing wrong with me is I have high cholesterol." But, and this should be underlined, in traditional medical circles a **problem** is usually not viewed as a significant problem until the constellation of symptoms and signs meets the requirement designated by a name listed in standard medical classification directories (e.g. cancer, arthritis, etc.). Finally, **problems** may be viewed in bizarre ways. "Everything's fine except my financial health" or "It sure would be nice to work in a healthy place."

In the forthcoming chapters, we'll examine **problems** variously defined but having in common that they all suggest an unsolved issue. We'll start with one of America's biggest **problems**, namely tiredness.

2

ARE YOU AS BUSHED (AS MOST PEOPLE THINK THEY ARE)?

"I don't know why I'm so tired all the time. I go to bed exhausted and can hardly tear myself out in the morning. The doctor says there's nothing wrong with me. Then why can't I muster up the energy to do the things I used to really enjoy?"

* * *

That same question is being asked by men and women in thousands of offices, homes and factories everyday.

Tired...bushed...worn out...exhausted...weary...

these are but a few of the many synonyms for fatigue.

According to a recent Department of Health and Human Services report entitled **Reasons for Visiting Physicians**, a staggering 14 million Americans go to their doctor complaining of fatigue. Add to that uncounted millions who seek medical advice for other reasons but also mention significant exhaustion. And add to that, millions more who never seek help but are nonetheless tired all the time. It becomes clear that fatigue is a major problem in America!

Just what is it that's sapping the energy and drive from so many? For years medicine has pointed the finger at anemia, the inadequate consumption or loss of iron, as being the major cause of fatigue in women. None can argue that many females lose this element during cases of periodic menstrual bleeding. But, **iron poor blood** as the Madison Avenue advertisers who sell Geritol and Fem-Iron label it, isn't the only (and may not be the most important) causative agent that contributes to fatigue. When you get right down to it, exhaustion can strike anyone.

For the moment, back to the women, researchers in Sweden compared anemic females in the 38 to 60 age range with a non-anemic group who had similar sleeping habits, physical activity and histories of infectious diseases. They found no difference in weariness. It's true that more females than males complain of exhaustion, but most references in the medical literature make no bones about the fact that large numbers of men are equally afflicted.

The majority of researchers now agree that fatigue is multicausal, thus many factors, either singly or in combination can be at the root of the problem. These contributing factors range from the obvious such as poor sleeping habits, to others as diverse as smoking to having a boring job.

Identifying those areas in one's life—physical, social, and psychologic—which have been shown to contribute to symptoms of fatigue, is the only real way to start working on the problem. That's what this chapter is all about.

With the magnitude of this issue, one might expect that there are many questionnaires...and so it is...some are very simple; others complex.

Just for starters, we want you to complete two very simple forms. The first was developed by G. W. McNelly with variations by H. Yoshitake. Parenthetic mention should be made that Dr. Yoshitake reported his work from the Institute of Science and Labor in Tokyo, Japan. The second quiz was designed by the Industrial Fatigue Research Committee of the Japanese Association of Industrial Health. We gratefully acknowledge the permission by Doctors McNeely and Yoshitake and the Japanese Association of Industrial Health for allowing us the use of these materials.

Begin now by checking which one of the following best describes how you feel most of the time.

1. terrific ☐

2. very good ☐

3. energetic ☐

4. fairly well ☐

5. average ☐

6. a little tired ☐

7. dragging ☐

8. exhausted ☐

9. about to collapse ☐

In the box below put the number of the item you have checked which best describes you:

☐

If you've listed one of the numbers between 6 and 9, then you have some measure of chronic tiredness. Obviously, it would be highly desirable to reach something lower, possibly in the range of 3 to 5.

Should you wish a more sophisticated scoring of your exhaustion, there are many measuring forms available. As but one example, now turn your attention to the more quantitative fatigue test which consists of the next thirty questions.

Note the scoring system:
    0 = never
    1 = sometimes
    2 = frequently
    3 - usually
Put the number in the appropriate box.

1. Do you feel burning or heaviness in the head? ☐

2. Does your entire body feel tired? ☐

3. Do you feel as though you would like to lie down? ☐

4. Do your legs feel tired? ☐

5. Do your thoughts get confused or muddled? ☐

6. Are you drowsy? ☐

7. Do you yawn a lot? ☐

8. Are your eyes tired? ☐

9. Do you have trouble moving? ☐

10. Do you feel dizzy or have trouble standing? ☐

11. Do you have difficulty concentrating? ☐

12. Do you get tired of talking? ☐

13. Are you nervous? ☐

14. Do you forget things? ☐

15. Do you feel a lack of self-confidence? ☐

16. Do you have difficulty standing or sitting up straight? ☐

17. Do you have difficulty thinking clearly? ☐

18. Does your attention wander easily? ☐

19. Do you become anxious easily? ☐

20. Do you find that your patience is short? ☐

21. Do you have a headache? ☐

22. Do you feel stiff in the shoulders? ☐

23. Do you feel a pain in the abdomen? ☐

24. Do you have trouble breathing? ☐

25. Do you feel thirsty? ☐

26. Does your voice sound husky? ☐

27. Are you dizzy? ☐

28. Do your eyelids twitch? ☐

29. Do you have shaking in the arms or legs? ☐

30. Do you feel nauseated? ☐

Add up the numbers to calculate your final score which is to be inserted in the box below:

☐

If your entire score on this examination lies between 0 and 30, you're lucky to be experiencing very little tiredness. Should the total range be between 31 and 60 then there's evidence of a moderate amount of fatigue. If your overall grade is 60 or more, then you're one of those many people with a real problem.

Tiredness...exhaustion...fatigue...there are literally tens of other analogues such as ennui...boredom. The hottest and newest twentieth century cliché is burnout.

Doctor Herbert J. Freudenberger has captured

eloquently this so-called new syndrome: "If you have ever seen a building that has been burned out, you know it's a devastating sight. What had once been a throbbing, vital structure is now deserted. Where there had once been activity, there are now only crumbling reminders of energy and life. Some bricks or concrete may be left; some outlines of windows. Indeed, the outer shell may seem almost intact. Only if you venture inside will you be struck by the full force of the desolation."

It's for sure that people like buildings can burnout. The complex world we live in imposes such extraordinary demands on our inner resources that the burnout syndrome is devastating literally millions of American workers, leaving them a mere shell of their former selves. It's, unfortunately, often an occupational hazard that strikes the best and the brightest. Look upon it as a smoldering fire that smothers ambition, relationships, health and happiness by inevitably stiffling the very energy that fuels high achievers.

Historically implied (and this has been pointed out earlier) is that fatigue is a special female problem due to low iron. The more contemporary thinking, as has already been mentioned earlier in this chapter, is that tiredness is usually a physical disorder which is the result of poor lifestyle. Suggested now in this just-described account of burnout is that it's principally or exclusively a mental or emotional state.

The fact of the matter is that, however named... fatigue or burnout, the result is the same or similar. This will become evident as we'll see in the forthcoming questionnaire.

The following form was developed by Dr. Herbert J. Freudenberger. We wish to take this opportunity to thank him for granting us permission to reproduce his questionnaire. He proposes you examine the past few months for changes in your lifestyle. Allow yourself about 30 seconds to answer each question. Assign a number from one, representing no or little change, to five for a major change.

1. Do you tire more easily? Feel fatigued rather than energetic?

2. Are people annoying you by telling you "You don't look so good lately"?

3. Are you working harder and harder and accomplishing less and less?

4. Are you increasingly cynical and disenchanted?

5. Are you often invaded by a sadness you can't explain?

6. Are you forgetting appointments, deadlines, personal possessions?

7. Are you increasingly irritable? More short-tempered? More disappointed in the people around you?

8. Are you seeing close friends and family members less frequently?

9. Are you too busy to do even routine things like make phone calls or read reports or send out birthday cards?

10. Are you suffering from physical complaints (aches, pains, head aches, a lingering cold)? ☐

11. Do you feel disoriented when the activity of the day comes to a halt? ☐

12. Is joy elusive? ☐

13. Are you unable to laugh at a joke about yourself? ☐

14. Does sex seem like more trouble than it's worth? ☐

15. Do you have very little to say to people? ☐

Now add up your score and insert in the box.

☐

The lowest possible score is 15; the highest attainable is 75. How did you do and what does it mean?

From zero to 25, you're doing just fine. Twenty-six to 35 may be a signal to keep your eye out. With a grade between 36 and 50, you're a candidate for burnout. And, for sure, if your grade is between 51 and 65 you really have a problem. Over 65, beware! You're in a dangerous position that is threatening your physical and mental wellbeing.

Remember, these numbers are not **holy**, the demarcation lines between the groups are arbitrary. Also, keep in mind the good news...luckily burnout or near-burnout is reversible.

Where do you begin?

According to Dennis T. Jaffe and Cynthia Scott,

in their superb **From Burnout to Balance: A workbook for Peak Performance and Self-Renewal**, there are two key concepts in coping with inordinate stress. The first is to sort out what you can change and what you cannot. Secondly, to decide where to place your effort and energy. Clearly, it's smart to begin by modifying what you can control. Choosing the other is the fast-track to inevitable and ceaseless burnout.

As a matter of fact, for those who score in the marginal ranges, the warning zones, a good place to begin is to refer to the Scott/Jaffe Book (p. 33).

It should be emphasized that not every personality is subject to burnout. Surely, it would be highly unlikely, if not impossible, for the underachiever to get into this potential state. The happy-go-lucky soul with modest aspirations is not a candidate either. This syndrome is reserved for the dynamic, the charismatic, the goal-oriented man or woman who want and strive for the **best**—the **best** marriage, the **best** job, the **best** child, the **best** of everything!

Reading books and articles is just fine for those without burnout and for those with some early and relatively benign manifestations of the syndrome. But for those who scored significantly on the questionnaire, much more is needed immediately.

Now is the place and the time for professional assistance which may take the form of a friend, a pastor, a psychologist, sometimes even experts in seemingly unrelated areas like a nutritional or physical fitness trainer. There are a number of places you can start looking for help. For example, you may wish to contact the American Association of Fitness Directors in Business and Industry, 400 Sixth Street, S. W., Washington, D. C. 20201. This is a membership organization of health promotion and stress management practitioners.

The Center for Health Promotion and Education at the Centers for Disease Control, Atlanta, Georgia 30333, provides technical assistance, publishes research, and helps in creating stress and health programs, and disseminates a large number of pertinent monographs.

And finally, there is the Washington Business Group on Health, 229½ Pennsylvania Avenue, S. E., Washington, D. C. 20003 (202-547-6644), which is a national organization of corporations that provides resources and information about health promotion, including burnout.

It's clear from this discussion that, in many instances, help is desirable or essential. Before one reaches out for such assistance, it might be well to ascertain what kind of counsel is appropriate. We'd suggest that you examine Part C of this book which deals with solutions. For instance, the fatigue/burnout syndrome identified in this chapter may have a large and significant dietary component. To quantify the eating habits, we would suggest that you read and answer the questionnaire(s) in that particular chapter. On the other hand, should it appear that smoking or alcohol consumption are dominant contributors to exhaustion, then clearly one should next check those appropriate sections. Finally, more particulars about the overall problem of stress is detailed in Chapter 8.

For the moment, we've looked at America's most common symptom. Obviously, there are others for which time and space are not being alloted here. If you're just interested in symptoms, there are others. Depression, probably America's number one mental complaint will be examined (Chapter 11).

RESOURCES

1. Atkinson, H.
   Women and Fatigue
   1985. New York, G. P. Putnam's Sons.

   This is a truly unique book for a number of reasons and especially because of the arrangement of questionnaires. Most of them modified by the author from others. It's also of interest as it makes available quiz forms to measure in a reasonably quantitative way the factors contributing to tiredness.

2. Basta, S. S., Karyadi, D. and Scrimshaw, N. S.
   Iron Deficiency Anemia and the Productivity of Adult Males in Indonesia.
   American Journal of Clinical Nutrition 32: #4, 916-925, April 1979.

   Approximately 88 percent of adult male workers on a rubber plantation in West Java (Indonesia) suffered with hookworm infestation and over 45 % were anemic as judged by hemoglobin below 13 grams. Hemoglobin values and performance as measured by the Harvard Step Test (HST) for both tappers and weeders were significantly correlated. The rubber tappers were paid by their work output and their earnings correlated with hemoglobin levels. Treatment with 100 milligrams of elemental iron for 60 days resulted in a significant improvement in hematologic status of the anemic individuals and in their performance, work output, and morbidity.

3. Cheraskin, E., Ringsdorf, W. M., Jr., and Medford, F. H.
Daily Vitamin C Consumption and Fatigability
Journal of the American Geriatrics Society 24: #3, 136-137, March 1976.

It has long been known, actually since about 1750, that sailors on long voyages frequently suffered with inordinate fatigue. For this and other reasons, 411 dental practitioners were queried by a simple seven-point questionnaire regarding tiredness. Additionally, vitamin C consumption by means of a simple food frequency questionnaire was ascertained. It was discovered that the 81 subjects who consumed less than 100 milligrams of vitamin C per day recorded a fatigability score approximately twice that of the 330 subjects who ingested more than 400 milligrams of vitamin C on a daily basis.

4. Cheraskin, E. Ringsdorf, W. M., Jr. and Sisley, E. L.
The Vitamin C Connection
1983. New York, Harper & Row Publishers, Inc. (hardback).
1984. New York, Bantam Books, Inc. p. 135-145 (paperback).

This book, written for lay-educational purposes, includes a chapter on **tired blood**. It is noteworthy for several reasons. Firstly, there's an abbreviated seven-question form extracted from the time-honored and tested Cornell Medical Index Health Questionnaire. Secondly, this chapter shows unequivocally the overall relationship between ascorbic acid and fatigability. Finally, there is an appended bibliography of support data.

5. Cypress, B. K.
Patients' Reasons for Visiting Physicians: National Ambulatory Medical Care Survey.
1981. Hyattsville, Maryland, United States Department of Health and Human Services, DHHS Publication No. (PHS) 82-1717.

This report presents a detailed tabular analysis of data collected in the National Ambulatory Medical Care Survey (NAMCS) of the National Center for Health Statistics on patient's reasons for visiting office-based physicians, determined from a classification system developed in 1977 for use in this survey.

Data collection and processing for the 1977 and 1978 NAMCS were the responsibility of the University of Chicago's National Opinion Research Center. Sample selection was accomplished with the assistance of the American Medical Association (AMA) and the American Osteopathic Association (AOA).

The evidence suggests that approximately 14,000,000 persons presented a primary complaint of tiredness/exhaustion/weakness.

6. Ellis, F. R. and Nasser, S.
   A Pilot Study of Vitamin B$_{12}$ in the Treatment of Tiredness
   British Journal of Nutrition 30: #2, 277-283, September 1973.

   Twenty-eight subjects complaining of tiredness completed a doubleblind cross-over trial of injections of vitamin B$_{12}$ (5 milligrams twice weekly for two weeks) followed by a rest period of two weeks and then a similar course of matching placebo injections. Symptoms were assessed by a daily self-rating method and included appetite, mood, energy, sleep, and general feeling of well being. The principal conclusion is that there was significant improvement (reduction) in tiredness with vitamin B$_{12}$ administration.

7. Freudenberger, H. J. and Richelson, G.
   Burn Out: How to Beat the High Cost of High Achievement
   1980. New York, Doubleday and Company.

   The senior author is a practicing psychoanalyst who developed the last questionnaire in this chapter. Among his many worthwhile points, is how to check burnout at, or before, its onset. There are many exciting chapters including, for example, the subjects of exhaustion, detachment and boredom.

8. Jaffe, D. T. and Scott, C.
   From Burnout to Balance: A Workbook for Peak Performance and Self-Renewal

1984. New York, McGraw Hill Book Company.

Doctors Jaffe and Scott are management consultants and clinical psychologists who design programs on burnout, health promotion and peak performance for many organizations. The central theme of their book is that in our present complex and demanding world people must learn to manage, maintain and renew themselves. These skills are as essential to self-preservation and effective work performance and survival as the customary and traditional skills of managing other people and resources. This workbook is designed to help you respond creatively to the diverse pressures and demands of your work and your life.

9. McDonagh, E. W., Rudolph, C. J. and Cheraskin, E.
The Effect of EDTA Chelation Therapy with Multivitamin/Trace Mineral Supplementation Upon Reported Fatigue
Journal of Orthomolecular Psychiatry 13: #4, 277-279, Fourth Quarter 1984.

More often than not, in this paper as well as in common parlance, diet and nutrition are viewed interchangeably. Strictly speaking, this is not true. More precisely, diet represents what one eats; nutrition encompasses what nutrients reach their termination as a function of absorption, assimilation, utilization and excretion. Simply put, one may "eat well" and still be malnourished. This report underlines that distinction. Specifically, 139 private patients were studied in terms of fatigability before and after a series of chelation infusions. The evidence suggest that, under these presumably improved nutritional conditions, fatigability was reduced approximately 39%.

10. McNelly, G. W.
The Development and Laboratory Validation of Subjective Fatigue Scale
In Tiffin, J. and McCormick, E. J.
Industrial Psychology
1966. London, George Allen & Unwin Ltd.

This investigator, resulting from his doctoral dissertation, provides us with a very simple and reasonably sensitive measure of fatigue based on nine questions judged very reliably in terms of subjective tiredness.

11. Medical News
Low Potassium May Weaken Grip in the Aged, Study in Scotland Suggests
Journal of the American Medical Association 210: #1, 25, 6 October 1969.

At least some of the muscular weakness usually attributed to aging may actually be due to a dietary deficiency of potassium according to a report by two investigators from the University of Glasgow. In their study muscular strength was measured by right hand grip pressure and was found to decrease with lower potassium consumption. Sixty percent of the women and approximately forty percent of the men in the group were deemed to not be getting an adequate amount of potassium in the diet. Those with the deficiency had a significantly weaker grip pressure than normal for people of the same age, sex, and weight.

12. Paine, W. S.
Job Stress and Burnout: Research, Theory, and Intervention Perspectives
1982. Beverly Hills, Sage Publications.

Almost every major pioneer in the area of burnout research is represented in this volume. Much of the material contained in this 295 page book emerged from the First National Conference on Burnout held in Philadelphia in 1981. This is a scholarly piece of work, and could prove to be a valuable resource, particularly to individuals concerned with burn-out syndrome in an organizational setting.

13. Poleliakhoff, A.
Adrenocortical Activity and Some Clinical Findings in Acute and Chronic Fatigue
Journal of Psychosomatic Research 25: #2, 91-95, 1981.

Hormonal changes, notably plasma cortisol levels, were significantly lower in a group of patients suffering with chronic fatigue as compared to an age and sex matched control group. Additionally, social readjustment rating scores were also significantly higher in the exhaustion subset. Here's an excellent example of an established relationship between fatigability and hormonal activity.

14. Ray, M. B.
    How Never to be Tired: or Two Lifetimes in One
    1983. New York, The Bobbs-Merrill Company, Inc.

    This book presents an open—and—shut case for the theory that fatigue and boredom are closely allied and that people grow weary less readily when doing things they like. It was first published in 1938. In 1944, it was revised. Now, in its present form, this popular treatise on fatigue has been praised by outstanding psychiatrists as the best lay presentation of the causes and cure of fatigue ever written.

15. Vigderman, P.
    Coping With Burnout: How to Feed the Fire of your Ambition Without Letting Your Life go up in Smoke.
    New Age Journal 46-51, August 1985.

    Burnout is not a disease, nor is it the inevitable consequence of a job loaded with stressors. The author contends that "the very talents that lead to a high-pressure position, such as quick thinking, flexibility, and self-confidence, can be called on to prevent a person's sense of well-being from going up in flames." Authorities on burnout offer advice on ways to recognize, cope with, and reverse the syndrome. This informative article also covers such diverse areas as managing the boss, time management, creativity under pressure, and tips on exercise to reduce stress. The questionnaire used in this chapter of Health and Happiness (from Dr. Herbert J. Freudenberger's book Burn Out: How to Beat the High Cost of High Achievement) is included.

16. Welch, I. D., Medeiros, D. C. and Tate, G. A.
Beyond Burnout: How to Enjoy Your Job Again When You've Just About Had Enough
1982. Englewood Cliffs, Prentice-Hall, Inc.

While more studies on burnout are being completed, and more books written on the subject, few are as comprehensive and easy to read as this excellent resource. The authors discovered five areas of human functioning that are affected by burnout namely, the physical, intellectual, emotional, social, and spiritual. Each chapter in the text is divided into three sections which deal with causes, symptoms, and suggestions for prevention or relief. The primary assumption which underlines this book is that people are responsible for their own burnout. Somewhere in their lives they have made decisions which facilitate burnout. To the extent that this is true, they are free to change those decisions and reverse the process. Numerous self administered, self-graded questionnaires are scattered throughout the book.

17. Yoshitake, H.
Relations Between the Symptoms and the

Feeling of Fatigue
Ergonomics 14: #1, 175-186, January 1971.

There are many fatigue questionnaires. The one developed by this investigator, based on his experience in industry (broadcasters and bank clerks) is cited in the text for completion by the readership. It's noteworthy that there seems to be an almost linear relationship between feelings and complaints of fatigue.

3

ARE YOU GOING TO GET CANCER?

As we've discovered in the last chapter, to some a **problem** connotes a symptom or a sign. For that reason plus its popularity, we initiated this section on **problems** with fatigue. Incidentally, we'll return with another common symptom depression in Chapter 11—Other Problems.

To others, especially in the scientific community, a **problem** means a discrete **disease**. In other words, more often than not, doctors view problems as arthritis, diabetes and heart disease. For sure, a big **problem** is cancer. True, it's not as popular as fatigue but what it lacks in commonness, it makes up in seriousness.

Part of the reason why cancer is so complex stems from the jaw-breaking mantle of mumbo-jumbo. So, let's begin with a clarification of lingo. For sure, the buzz-word **cancer** makes the purists shudder. The oncologists (cancer specialists) are wedded to a very detailed and descriptive classification of tumors based upon the site of origin, the degree of malignancy, and the life-threatening potential. Some of the lines of demarcation are as fuzzy as the distinction between liberal Republicans and conservative Democrats. For our purposes, as well as the American Cancer Society, **cancer** signifies any life-threatening tumor.

Here's the bad news...

- According to some authoritative estimates, about one in four in this country, meaning approximately 56 million red-blooded Americans, will eventually suffer with cancer.
- This is another way of saying that two out of every three families will be tragically touched.
- The decade of the 1970s saw an incidence increase of between five and ten percent.
- In the 1980s, a thousand people die daily from a melanoma type skin cancer. This translates into one death every 78 seconds.

That's the bad news.

The good news is that there is increasing and comforting evidence that environmental factors, notably tobacco and diet are believed to contribute to as much as 90 percent of all human cancer in the United States (Ref. 1, p. 47).

In plain English, we can prevent cancer!

More specifically, researchers now hold that

approximately 60 percent of cancer in women and 40 percent of malignant growths in men may well be the result in part, for example, of eating habits. (For this, as well as other reasons, you'll note in future chapters the role of diet as a solution to many problems.)

Now is the time to evaluate your overall risk for cancer. The following simple eight-question test was developed by one of the prestigious cancer organizations (reprinted with permission from the American Institute of Cancer Research).

Now to the questionnaire. Choose only one response in each category that most closely matches your lifestyle. After reading each statement, mark (in the space provided) the number of points (shown in parentheses) that corresponds with your answer.

weight
- a) ideal weight for build (0)
- b) twenty percent or more above ideal weight (3)
- c) twenty percent or more below ideal weight (1)

diet
- a) consume thirty percent or less of calories from fats; eat vegetables and whole grains regularly (0)
- b) eat fatty meats, fried foods, high fat dairy products and sweets three times a week (2)
- c) eat fatty meats, fried foods, high fat dairy products and sweets daily (4)

smoking

- a) never smoked (0)
- b) smoke occasionally (4)
- c) quit smoking after smoking one-two packs a day for less than ten years (4)
- d) quit smoking after smoking one-two packs a day for more than ten years (5)
- e) now smoke one or more packs a day and have smoked for more than ten years (8)

alcohol
- a) don't drink, or consume fewer than six drinks a week (0)
- b) drink to the point of getting high or drunk two or more times a week (1)
- c) drink to the point of getting high or drunk four or more times a week (3)

stress
- a) rarely feel harried; have no trouble relaxing (0)
- b) feel really under pressure three/four times in a typical week (1)
- c) almost always seem pressured or harried; have great difficulty relaxing (2)

sleep
- a) no trouble getting to sleep; wake up refreshed (0)
- b) have some trouble falling

asleep and staying asleep, but usually wake up refreshed (1)
c) frequently have difficulty sleeping and often wake up tired (2)
d) no trouble falling asleep but wake up tired (1)

physical activity
a) get vigorous exercise at least three times a week for at least thirty minutes (0)
b) lead active life but don't exercise (1)
c) have sedentary lifestyle (3)

medical examinations
a) have medical check-ups and screenings (such as pap tests, breast self-examinations) at recommended intervals (0)
b) have medical check-ups and screenings sporadically, but pay close attention to early warning signs (2)
c) only see a doctor when sick (4)

total

Now to the tally.

If your score is 0 to 5, you have a healthy lifestyle. It's unlikely your present habits will invite cancer.

Should the sum be 6 to 10 you also lead a fairly healthy life, but you have at least one negative risk factor.

A range of 11 to 15 exposes several risk elements.

A grade of 16 to 20 means you have a higher-than-average risk of developing cancer (and incidentally other chronic diseases). Obviously, eliminating these can only be beneficial.

Finally, with a score of 21 to 29, your lifestyle is killing you! See a health practitioner to identify ways for reducing your very high risk for cancer and other life-threatening diseases.

Clearly, this simple questionnaire is designed to provide simple answers. There are many other cancer forms more complicated but allow more detailed information. For more data, consult the Resource Section of this chapter.

The final story on cancer has obviously not been written. The picture, as we've already indicated, is still grim. The question which remains is why after great expenditures of time, money, and energy, the problem has not been solved.

There are reasons understandable if not good.

The prevailing cancer concept holds that we're dealing with a **specific** set of syndromes (e.g. squamous cell carcinoma, Kaposi's sarcoma, mesothioloma) for which there are **specific** therapeutic modalities (e.g. surgery, radiation, chemotherapy). The truth of the matter is that cancer is actually a collection of **nonspecific** syndromes (e.g. best viewed as carcinomatosis) for which there are **nonspecific** answers (e.g. diet, physical activity, clean air).

This hypothesis must be correct. As but one example, the real success with lung cancer didn't follow innovations in surgery, radiation, or chemotherapy. The **real** successes appeared with the reduction in tobacco consumption.

In other words, the real answer to cancer will come with techniques which make possible **primary prevention** (prevention of occurrence). These tools are only given lip service in traditional circles. For example, mammography, sigmoidoscopy, pap smears and other such procedures don't really constitute primary prevention. They should, of course, be applauded because they provide **secondary prevention** (prevention of recurrence) or early detection. But they don't contribute to primary prevention (prevention of occurrence).

The hard evidence that these statements are correct are once again borne out by the great successes of lowered tobacco intake in lung cancer.

It should, therefore, follow that now is the time to examine your own lifestyle. If the answers in the questionnaire in this chapter were incomplete or not convincing, then it would be well to turn to Section C Solutions for clarification and confirmation.

In the meanwhile, more detailed information regarding lifestyle and cancer is provided in some of the abstracts which appear in the bibliographic material at the end of this chapter. You'll find, for example, exciting evidence of diet (folic acid) and cervical cancer (p. 48); sugar and vitamin C in carcinomatosis (p. 49).

RESOURCES

1. Alabaster, O.
   The Power of Prevention
   1985. New York, Simon & Schuster

   This highly readable and revealing book emphasizes the fact that environmental elements, notably tobacco and diet, are believed to contribute to as much as 90 percent of all human cancer in the United States. This underscores the incontestable fact that cancer is indeed a preventable problem.

Clearly, in the light of these figures, we must now look harder at the role of diet in cancer. This book uniquely sets out and accomplishes this goal.

Doctor Alabaster makes the very cogent point that since more than a quarter of the total population will eventually develop cancer, this means that about 60 million Americans will be affected. Of these, approximately 20 million cases might be prevented by relatively simple changes in the national diet!

2. American Institute for Cancer Research
   What's Your risk of Cancer?
   Lifestyle 406, Summer 1986.

   As but one example of the diversity of cancer questionnaires, this bulletin includes a 29-question form (in contrast to the eight-question test in this chapter). Clearly, this is an example of a more detailed interrogatory and, as one might expect, provides more specific cancer risk information.

3. Butterworth, C. E., Jr., Hatch, K. D., Gore, H., Mueller, H. and Krumdieck, C. L.
   Improvement in Cervical Dysplasia Associated with Folic Acid Therapy in Users of Oral Contraceptives
   American Journal of Clinical Nutrition 35: #1, 73-82, January 1982.

Forty-seven young women with mild or moderate dysplasia of the uterine cervix diagnosed by cervical smears, received oral supplements of folic acid or a placebo daily for three months under double blind conditions. All had used a contraceptive agent for six months. Biopsy scores from folate supplemented subjects were significantly better than in folate-unsupplemented women. These studies unearth two possibilities. First, it suggests a potential reversible localized derangement in folate metabolism which may sometimes be misdiagnosed as cervical dysplasia. Secondly, the experiment demonstrates an imbalance in the integral component of the dysplastic process that may be arrested or in some cases reversed by oral folic acid supplementation.

4. Cameron, E. and Pauling, L.
    Cancer and Vitamin C
    1979. New York, W. W. Norton and Company.

When this text hit the book stores in 1979, it created quite a stir in the medical community. While researchers were wary of a vitamin C cancer connection, they could not dispute the credibility of Dr. Pauling, a two-time Nobel Prize winner, and Dr. Cameron, a well respected Scottish researcher who has received many awards in pathology and medicine. The authors discuss in detail the nature, causes, prevention and treatment of cancer, while emphasizing the value of vitamin C as a supportive measure. They confirm their claims of ascorbic acid's value by detailing the accounts of more than 50 cancer patients who, in varying degress, benefitted from its use as an adjunct therapy. The text, however, goes far beyond vitamin C. Drs. Pauling and Cameron also weigh the limitations and value of various accepted procedures in the treatment of cancer, including chemotherapy, immunotherapy, hormones, and unorthodox modalities.

5. Cheraskin, E., and Ringsdorf, W. M., Jr.
Carbohydrate Metabolism and Carcinomatosis
Cancer 17: #2, 159-162, February 1964.

During the past three quarters of a century, numerous reports linking carbohydrate metabolism and carcinomatosis have appeared in the literature. In general, the observations have been based on the study of the frequency of diabetes-like disease in cancer patients and the occurrence of malignant tumors in individuals with diabetes-like disease. This study was designed to investigate the pattern of carbohydrate metabolism in two groups of noncancer subjects, one with and one without a positive familial cancer background. Forty age-paired noncancer firemen and policemen were selected from 100 volunteers on the basis of a positive (20 subjects) or negative (20 subjects) familial history of cancer. Blood sugar and glucose levels revealed a significantly greater variance in the subjects with a positive oncologic history meaning greater dysglycemia (both hyper- and hypoglycemia).

6. Cheraskin, E., Ringsdorf, W. M., Jr., Hutchins, K., Setyaadmadja, A. T. S. H. and Wideman, G. L.
   Carbohydrate Metabolism and Cervical (Uterine) Carcinoma
   American Journal of Obstetrics and Gynecology 97: #6, 817-820, 15 March 1967.

   The classical glucose tolerance test was performed on 26 ambulatory, nonhospitalized, biopsy-proved squamous cell cervical carcinoma patients and compared with similar testing of 26 age- and sex-paired individuals without cancer. Three items deserve special mention. First, the frequency of glycosuria (sugar in the urine) in the cancer group is approximately fourfold that observed in the noncancer subset. Second, the frequency of elevated blood glucose levels in the cancer category is approximately twofold that in the noncancer group. Third, the mean blood glucose values at every temporal point are statistically higher in the oncologic group versus those without cancer.

7. Cheraskin, E., Ringsdorf, W. M., Jr., and Clark, J. W.
   Diet and Disease
   1968. Emmaus, Rodale Press, Inc. (hardback)
   1977. New Canaan, Keats Publishing Co. (paperback)

   The authors offer a well researched, detailed analysis of the American diet and its relationship to a variety of diseases, including cancer. Using evidence from medical laboratories around the world, these investigators strongly suggest that the role of diet as a factor in the development of cancer and other diseases which afflict Americans is grossly underestimated. Studies completed subsequent to the publication of the text have borne this out. Even the National Cancer Institute and the American Cancer Society now acknowledge a link between certain forms of the disease and diet. For those interested in a scholarly approach to the subject, Diet and Disease is an adequate primer.

8. Cheraskin, E. Ringsdorf, W. M., Jr., Setyaadmadja, A. T. S. H., Barrett, R. A., Aspray, D. W. and Curry, S.
Cancer Proneness Profile: A Study in Weight and Blood Glucose
Geratrics 23: #4, 134-137, April 1968.

Capillary blood glucose (Dextrostix method) two to four hours after food or drink or both were consumed was determined in 517 participants of the Birmingham, Alabama, Diabetes Detection Drive. The blood glucose scores were compared with the reported incidence of overweight and cancer by means of a self-administered questionnaire. The data suggest that, with advancing age, subjects with blood glucose scores of 80 to 95 mg. percent report more cancer than individuals with blood glucose values in the 60 to 75 mg. percent range. The results suggest that, in older people, those who are overweight report more cancer than those who deny obesity. Within the limits of these observations, individuals with slightly higher blood glucose levels report more cancer than when these two variables are considered separately.

9. Cheraskin, E., Ringsdorf, W. M., Jr. Hutchings, K., Setyaadmadja, A. T. S. H. and Wideman, G.
Effect of Diet upon Radiation Response in Cervical Carcinoma of the Uterus: A Preliminary Report
Acta Cytologica 12: #6, 433-438, November-December 1968.

The radiation response was studied in 54 female subjects with biopsy-proven squamous cell carcinoma of the uterine cervix. Twenty-seven underwent nutritional therapy prior to irradiation; the remaining 27 served as controls. The radiation response is significantly higher following dietary changes than observed under control conditions.

10. Cheraskin, E., Ringsdorf, W. M., Jr., and Aspray, D. W.
Cancer Proneness Profile: A Study in Ponderal Index and Blood Glucose
Geratrics 24: #8, 121-125, August 1969.

A study of 507 subjects shows a relationship between an anthropometric assessment of weight (ponderal index) and an estimate of carbohydrate metabolism (blood glucose by the Dextrostix method) versus the incidence of reported carcinomatosis. No cancer was observed in the 0 to 29 year age group, regardless of ponderal index or blood glucose levels. In the 30-

to 49-year old category, however a cancer incidence of 12.2% was noted in the obese subjects with lower glucose levels. In the older age subset (50+ years) 13.6% of the subjects reported cancer. These were essentially the overweight persons with relatively higher blood glucose levels.

11. Cheraskin, E., Ringsdorf, W. M., Jr. and Sisley, E. L.
The Vitamin C Connection
1983. New York, Harper & Row Publishers, Inc. (hardback)
1984. New York, Bantam Books, Inc. (paperback)

This lay text is designed to describe generally unknown connections between vitamin C and disease problems. Particularly relevant here is the fact that there's an entire chapter dealing with the relationship of ascorbic acid to malignant states. It's well to underline that, included in that particular chapter is a small questionnaire of 12 items intended to ascertain the possible vitamin C cancer interrelationship.

12. Creasey, W. A.
Diet and Cancer
1985. Philadelphia, Lea & Febiger.

This rather thorough work details what's known about the relationships between food and the incidence of various primary cancers. Using many references from the medical literature, Creasey examines the correlation between protein and caloric intake, dietary fiber, fats, vitamins and minerals. There's also a review of what's known about carcinogenicity and the consumption of alcohol and coffee. This book is an excellent resource for those wishing to know more about the nutrition/cancer link.

13. Greenwald, P. and Sondik, E. J.
    NCI Monographs
    1986. Bethesda, National Cancer Institute

    This report, which was prepared by the Division of Cancer Prevention and Control of the National Cancer Institute, is a thorough analysis and synthesis of current knowledge about the prevention and control of cancer through many avenues, particularly lifestyle factors, screening and treatment. The authors, drawn from a vast pool of the nation's most respected researchers, clinicians and public health specialists, flatly state "a reduction in the cancer mortality rate of as much as 50 percent is possible if current recommendations regarding smoking reduction, diet changes, screening, and state-of-the-art treatment are effectively applied." To the best of our knowledge, this is the most current appraisal of what must be done to slash deaths due to cancer.

14. Simonton, C. O., Simonton, S. M., and Creighton, J.
    Getting Well Again: A Step by Step Self-Help Guide to Overcoming Cancer for Patients and Their Families

1978. Los Angeles, Tarcher.

Around 1971, Carl O. Simonton of Dallas, started using mental imagery to treat patients with terminal cancer. Simonton had trained for three years to become a cancer specialist and he had seen dozens of patients use will-power and imagination to defy their doctors' grim prognoses.

Along with his former wife, who is a psychologist, he started showing how attitudes could alter the course of a disease. By 1978, when the Simontons published their best-selling Getting Well Again, they had trained 159 patients who had been branded incurable. Although all of their victims had been expected to die within a year of diagnosis, most survived for at least 20 months, and more than a quarter partially or completely recovered.

4

HOW'S YOUR ARTHRITIS?

As we've seen in the last chapter, it's for sure that cancer is a big and serious problem. It's also for certain that by time-tested and largely conventional means it can be treated. What's even more exciting is that there's increasing evidence that cancer can be prevented by simple lifestyle modifications.

Arthritis, while possibly not as deadly as cancer, is a big and crippling problem.

- **Arth** is the stem for joint and **itis** means inflammation. So strictly speaking, arthritis is supposed to signify inflammation of the

joints.
- Actually, there are over 100 different types of arthritis.
- Some are characterized by inflammation; others not. Some involve the joints; others the tissues surrounding the joints.
- It's estimated that 36 million Americans—from toddlers to centurions—suffer from some kind of arthritis.
- This does not include the millions that don't even know they have joint problems.
- For practical purposes, arthritis and rheumatism are synonymous.

In the everyday world, arthritis usually means one of two afflictions. One is osteoarthritis (OA) and the other is rheumatoid arthritis (RA).

The incidence of OA, also known as degenerative joint disease, far outweighs the rheumatoid variety. It's been around for centuries. Actually, it was discovered in mummies unearthed from Egyptian pyramids, and in the skeletal remains of other ancient civilizations. In the lower animal kingdom, even dinosaurs suffered from it. As a rule, OA is less crippling than rheumatoid arthritis, and older people are its most frequent victims. It's characterized by a degeneration of joint cartilage that cushions the ends of bones where they move against one another. As a result, the cartilage wears unevenly. When disability does occur, it's usually because of the disease's presence in weight bearing joints like the knees, hips and spine.

RA, on the other hand, is a chronic inflammatory syndrome that can affect 20 or more joints at one time. Other tissues may also be involved, including the lungs, spleen, skin and occasionally the heart. RA strikes all age groups and usually sets in somewhere between the years of 30 and 40; however, it's even been seen in babies as young as six months old. It's not uncommon for the symptoms of RA to go into remission, disappearing for a day, a month, or even years. Sometimes they never return.

If you have arthritis, and want to check how you're doing, the following questionnaire will help. Even if you haven't been diagnosed as suffering with a joint problem, take it anyway...you may be surprised. This quiz, from the authoritative book **Arthritis: A Comprehensive Guide,** by Dr. James Fries, is currently being used by many arthritis centers across the nation to evaluate the status of their patients. We want to acknowledge the permission granted to us for the use of this questionnaire. Armed with this valuable tool, anyone with arthritis can check their current status and their progress with time.

Use the following scale to grade the response that best describes your abilities as they usually are now for questions 1 through 8.

    0 = without difficulty
    1 = with difficulty
    2 = with help from another
    3 = unable to do at all

Write the appropriate number in the box following each statement.

Daily Function:

1. Dressing: Can you get your clothes, dress yourself, shampoo your hair...

2. Standing up: Are you able to stand up from a straight chair without

using your arms to push off... ☐

3. Eating: Can you cut your meat and lift a cup to your mouth... ☐

4. Walking: Can you walk outdoors on flat ground... ☐

5. Hygiene: Can you wash and dry your entire body, turn faucets, and get on and off the toilet... ☐

6. Reach: Can you reach up to and get down a seven-pound object that is above your head... ☐

7. Grip: Can you open push-button car doors and jars that have been previously opened... ☐

8. Activity: Can you drive a car or run errands and shop... ☐

For question 9, use the following chart.
    0 = without difficulty
    1 = somewhat painful or no sexual partner
    2 = very painful
    3 = impossible because of arthritis

Sexual Function:

9. Sex: Are you able to have sexual relations... ☐

The scoring system below is applicable for question 10:

0 = none
1 = mild
2 = moderate
3 = severe

Pain and Discomfort:

10. Severity: How would you describe the pain from your arthritis over the past week? ☐

Finally, for question number 11 use:
 0 = no pain
 1 = better
 2 = the same
 3 = worse

11. Trend: How has the severity of the pain changed over the past week? ☐

That's the test. Now, put the numbers (0, 1, 2, 3) corresponding to your answers in the appropriate spaces of the **arthritis rating sheet** that follows. It's essential that you answered all of the questions to have a valid score.

arthritis rating sheet

Daily Function:

1. dressing ☐

2. standing up ☐

3. eating ☐

4. walking ☐

5. hygiene ☐

6. reach ☐

7. grip ☐

8. activity ☐

9. sex ☐

Function points
(add 1 through 9) ☐

Pain and Discomfort:

10. severity ☐

11. trend ☐

Pain points
(add 10 and 11) ☐

How to interpret your score.

More than 500 patients at the Stanford Arthritis Center have taken the test you've just completed. They've all had arthritis for approximately 5 to 10 years. Compare your score to theirs to see how you match up.

Function points:

points	rating	percent of RA patients
0-4	normal	36%

5-13	adequate	47%
14-22	impaired	16%
23-27	disabled	1%

Pain points:

points	rating	percent of RA patients
0	none	2%
1-2	mild	8%
3-4	moderate	64%
5-6	severe	26%

Obviously, now you can decide whether you should seek additional assistance.

In the event that you're suffering with arthritis, two avenues are available.

With over 100 different types of arthritides one would expect many different therapies. And this is surely the case...with regard to the symptomatic management including physical therapy. But, the mainstay recommendations include pain control, gold injections and steroid therapy.

True, this regimen provides some measure of success in some subjects. For more particulars regarding such treatment modalities, you may wish to contact The Arthritis Foundation (AF), 1314 Spring Street, N.W., Atlanta, Georgia 30309, (404)872-7100. Founded in 1948, the AF is a national voluntary health association with 73 chapters that seeks the cause, prevention, and cure of arthritis. The AF works to help arthritis sufferers and their doctors through programs of research, patient services, health information, and professional education and training. There are AF chapters located in virtually every state that can provide you free literature pertaining to your particular form of rheumatic disease.

The University of Alabama at Birmingham Multipurpose Arthritis Center operates one of the nation's most comprehensive arthritis information services. The advice they provide is free and available to anyone in the country upon request. In addition, a monthly arthritis newsletter is offered free-of-charge. Write to the Arthritis Information Service, University of Alabama at Birmingham, 106 Basic Health Sciences Education and Research Building, Birmingham, Alabama 35294. Their fully trained counsellors will also field questions over the phone. Call (205)934-0542.

However, since the conventional results often leave much to be desired, it's not surprising that there's been an intensive search for other, more successful, and more simplistic options.

In general, the efforts have been directed at looking into lifestyle modifications. More specifically, the place of food, while controversial, is considered increasingly as a therapeutic alternative. Apropos, there are a number of studies, including one reported in the February 1986 issue of the prestigious British journal, The Lancet, that have shown the elimination of certain foods may benefit at least some patients (p. 67). The researchers, from the Department of Rheumatology at Epsom District Hospital in Surry, England, studied 49 rheumatoid arthritis patients. For one week all were given only well tolerated foods. They found that the frequency of pain during the day decreased from 36 to four percent. The average duration of morning stiffness was reduced from 53 to 10 minutes. Finally, the mean number of painful joints dropped from 22 to 18.

This study, and there are a number of others that make similar points, underlines the potential value of diet in the treatment of arthritis. The role of nutriture is heightened when one realizes that this hasn't been (and in most circles still isn't) part of orthodox medical practice. As but one piece of evidence, attention is directed to the bibliographic material and especially reference #1 cited from the Journal of the American Medical Association and published in 1935. You'll find in that abstract that at that time (and this thought still prevails unfortunately) diet is given no place in the treatment of arthritis.

If you want to explore in greater depth the role of your lifestyle as it relates to your joint problems, then turn to Part C: Solutions. This will allow you an opportunity to weigh your dietary habits, physical activity, tobacco and alcohol, and other social practices.

The big point is that there's help for arthritis. But this chapter (and especially when viewed in the light of the preceding one) makes an even bigger point. Most of us (including those in the medical professions) would never dream of viewing cancer and arthritis as the same or cousinly problems. Cancer is cancer. It's held to be a set of **specific** problems for which there are **specific** solutions. Arthritis is arthritis. It's generally viewed as a **specific** set of problems for which there's a **specific** set of solutions. Finally, conventional wisdom confirms that cancer and arthritis are clearly different problems.

But what we've discovered in these two chapters is that the traditional story may not be true. Cancer can be viewed as a **nonspecific** complex of problems for which we now know there are **nonspecific** answers. Likewise, it looks like arthritis can be judged a **nonspecific** matrix of disorders likely to be resolved by a **nonspecific** pattern of solutions. Finally, what's most exciting is the possibility that cancer and arthritis are really not all that different. At least, the solutions are very similar.

For the moment, you have two options. First, as we've indicated earlier, you can check your own lifestyle. Secondly, you might get some help by reviewing the appended bibliographic material.

RESOURCES

1. Bauer, W.
   What Should a Patient with Arthritis Eat?
   Journal of the American Medical Association 104: #1, 1-6, 5 January 1935.

   This report, published in America's most official medical journal, should be viewed in historical contexts. It makes the point back there in 1935 that, for practical purposes, diet plays little or no role in the management of most of the arthritides. This should be weighed against some of the more recent resources in this section showing the shift in thinking regarding diet and arthritis.

2. Berkley, G.
   Arthritis Without Aspirin
   1982. Englewood Cliff, Prentice-Hall, Inc.

   Professor Berkley from the University of Massachusetts has put together a book for lay-educational purposes. Its prime mission is to underline the nonpharmacalogic (orthomolecular) approach to the common arthritides. Special attention is assigned vitamins and minerals, water, light, physical activity and massage.

3. Cousins, N.
   Anatomy of an Illness
   1979. Toronto, W. W. Norton & Company

   The celebrated Norman Cousins (mentioned earlier in the chapter entitled Who's in Charge?) makes the point in this book that the solution to his devastating arthritic problem (ankylosing spondylitis) was made possible with a mixture of laughter and dietotherapy. The important point in his story is that he utilized treatment techniques not officially recognized by conventional authorities and resources.

4. Darlington, L. G., Ramsey, N. W., and Mansfield, J.R.
   Placebo-Controlled, Blind Study of Dietary Manipulation Therapy in Rheumatoid Arthritis
   Lancet 1: #8475, 236-238, 1 February 1986.

   A blind, placebo-controlled study of dietary manipulation therapy in 49 outpatients with rheumatoid arthritis disclosed a significant objective improvement during periods of dietary therapy compared with periods of placebo treatment. The percentage of patients with severe pain during the day decreased from 36 to 4 percent, average duration of morning stiffness reduced from 53 to 10 minutes, and the average number of painful joints reported dropped from

22 to 18. A blind clinical and laboratory assessment revealed significantly more improvement during the experimental versus the placebo period. The authors conclude dietary manipulation may benefit at least some patients with rheumatoid arthritis.

5. Fries, J.
   Arthritis: A Comprehensive Guide
   1979. Reading, Addison-Wesley Publishing Company

   Many experts consider this to be one of the best resources available to those suffering from arthritis. Dr. Fries, a highly respected physician and director of the Stanford Arthritis Clinic, answers most questions concerning the disease and the patient, including treatment, drugs, tests, biopsies, prevention, fatigue, weight loss, obesity, depression, pain, quackery, nausea, employment, and sexuality. Dr. Fries goes a step further than other authors by showing patients how to save money on medications, laboratory tests, x-rays, doctor visits, and hospitalization.

6. Hoffer, A.
   Treatment of Arthritis by Nicotinic Acid and Nicotinamide
   Canadian Medical Association Journal 81: #4, 235-238, 15 August 1959.

   The author, a psychiatrist, quite by accident discovered that the use of vitamin B_3 exerted salutary effects upon two of the common types of joint disease, namely rheumatoid and osteoarthritis. The publication of this information lead to a series of communications with Doctor William Kaufman who had earlier examined the role of niacin and niacinamide as a treatment for arthritis in several hundred subjects. The crux of this report includes the relating of the beneficial effects of vitamin B_3 in a small number of patients by the author. Also, there's an accounting of the earlier and extensive work by Doctor Kaufman showing the virtues of this vitamin singly and in combination with others in the arthritides.

7. Machtey, I. and Ouaknine, L.
Tocopherol in Osteoarthritis: A Controlled Pilot Study
Journal of the American Geriatrics Society 26: #7, 328-330, July 1978.

Thirty-two patients entered a simple-blind, cross-over study on the action of tocopherol in osteoarthritis. Each subject received either 600 milligrams alpha-tocopherol or a placebo for 10 days. The analgesic and other possible effects of tocopherol versus placebo were assessed by the patients' daily records and by the physicians' personal examination and interview. In 52 percent of the patients, a good tocopherol analgesic effect was noted.

8. McDonagh, E. W., Rudolph, C. J., and Cheraskin, E.
The "Clinical Change" in Patients Treated

with EDTA Chelation Plus Multivitamin/ Trace Mineral Supplementation.
Journal of Orthomolecular Psychiatry 14: #1, 61-65, First Quarter, 1985.

Traditionally, EDTA chelation is intended for the treatment of lead poisoning. This is a very interesting study of 139 patients, in a private practice environment, who underwent EDTA chelation. Additionally, system analysis was done by means of the Cornell Medical Index Health Questionnaire (CMI) before and after treatment. It was demonstrated that nonspecific musculosketal symptoms and signs were reduced by a magnitude of approximately 30%. This raises the possibility of favorably changing the arthritic state with improvement in circulation and possibly nutrition.

9. Reuler, J. B., Broudy, V. C. and Cooney, T. G.
Adult Scurvy
Journal of the American Medical Association 253: #36, 805-807, 8 February 1985.

It's now being recognized that scurvy, the classical expression of a vitamin C deficiency, can mimic many other medical syndromes. Three patients observed at the Oregon Health Sciences University and the Veterans Administration Medical Center in Portland, Oregon, with nonspecific muscle and joint pains were found, by dietary inquiry, to be lacking in vitamin C. Ascorbic acid supplementation reversed the pathologic process in all instances.

10. Warter, P. J., Crezner, H. L., Donio, D. A. and Horoschak, S.
Seven-Year Observations on the Treatment of Arthritis with Hesperidin-Ascorbic Acid
Journal of the American Geriatric Society 4: #6, 592-598, June 1956.

Long term observations are presented on (42) rheumatoid and (17) osteoarthritis patients, in whom hesperidin combined with ascorbic acid was used as a therapeutic adjuvant. It's demonstrated that this combination has the capacity to correct abnormal capillary fragility and permeability. The therapeutic management of arthritis is more effective in the presence of normal capillary resistance.

5

ARE YOU (LITERALLY) DYING TO BE THIN?

It's no secret in the publishing industry that there's big bucks in fat. From the most prestigious business journals to checkout counter tabloids, editors continue to innundate America with ways to shed the flab that stares back at us from the mirror. Are you (literally) dying to be fat?

- Adult Americans are 2.3 billion pounds over weight.
- The average American man weighs 4 pounds more than he did in 1960.
- The fattest Americans on average are black

women 45 to 74 years old; the skinniest is the elderly black male.
- The poor woman is most likely to be fat.
- In a study in the Boston area, overweight male high school seniors who had the same grades, IQ's, entrance-exam scores, and teachers' recommendations had only two-thirds the chance of being admitted to college than did their thinner counterparts.

The print and electronic media may be giving the country what it wants about the weight (meaning fat) problem. But there's a darker—even deadly—less-publicized side to an extreme preoccupation with underweight. It's called anorexia nervosa/bulimia.

Anorexia nervosa is the relentless pursuit of thinness and an overwhelming fear of becoming fat. Victims of this devastating disease actually starve themselves to achieve a thinness they perceive to be attractive. They constantly view themselves as fat and relentlessly strive to lose weight. It's pretty obvious, they're literally dying to be thin!
- Recent evidence suggest that 1/2 to 3 percent of the teenage population suffer with full-blown anorexia.
- One out of six may actually die.
- Usually it's found in upper class white girls.

The classical symptoms and signs of anorexia are fairly clearcut and hardly require a quiz or sophisticated diagnostic machinery to identify. The American Psychiatric Association's Diagnostic and Statistical Manual (DSM III), spells out the current criteria. The essential features of the disease include intense fear of becoming obese. The phobia doesn't diminish as more weight is lost. There's an obvious disturbance in body image, with patients claiming to feel fat even when they are emaciated. One encounters loss of more than 25 percent of original body weight. There's no known illness that could account for the weight loss. Finally, there can be the cessation or delay in onset of menstrual periods as a symptom. It's pretty obvious from this story how anorexia nervosa acquired it's psychiatric/psychologic classification.

One recent survey (1985), of 260 students at the University of California's Los Angeles campus, offers a glimpse of how widespread the fear of fat is, particularly among women. Better than 1 in 4 of the females in the survey said they were terrified of being fat. Only 5.8 percent of the men questioned fell into that category. On top of that, another approximately 1 in 4 of the coeds revealed they were obsessed or totally preoccupied with food compared to 7.5 percent of men. And 35 percent of the women said they felt fat, although others told them they were thin. Only 1 in 8 of the men believed they were obese despite others' contrary opinion.

Viewed in time, there's nothing new about anorexia nervosa. In the English language, reference to what is clearly anorexia can be traced back to medical writings of the 17th century. It says a lot for the abilities of those doctors that they recognized the syndrome as a fundamentally distinct entity amongst the welter of emaciating diseases of the times. But anorexia was not very fashionable until pop singer Karen Carpenter died following a long struggle with the disease.

Shortly after Karen's death, Jane Fonda, heralded for her famous fitness albums and video tapes, came forward to proclaim in print and on network television that from the age of 12 until she was 25 she was bulimic—binging and purging an incredible 15 to 20 times daily. It almost destroyed her.

Bulimia is not as well-known, but it too is a

devastating eating disorder. It's also a companion ailment to anorexia, since 25 to 60 percent of anorexics who do force themselves to eat indulge in purging.

Bulimia is new on the medical horizon. It was not recognized as a distinct and separate syndrome until 1980. It's characterized by an abnormal craving for food with resultant gorging. Then the victim either fasts, induces vomiting, or uses laxatives to purge the system.

Unlike anorexia, which usually strikes females, bulimia claims both men and women. Recent estimates show as many as 20 percent of adolescent and college age women are bulimic. One recent Gallup Poll, commissioned by the Comprehensive Care Corporation, reveals that of 504 teenagers surveyed, 40 percent of boys engaged in binge eating. A separate survey of 510 women uncovered that bulimia may well be affecting more than just adolescents.

An interesting observation about bulimia is that its victims are, almost without exception, young, white, in their twenties, from upper middle class families and with great potential. What is disconcerting is that the problem is now spreading to other groups.

Most bulimics are not obese, but many have had problems with compulsive eating and weight gain all their lives. They often swing from nutritionally unsound fad diets to food binges. When the diets don't work, they resort to purging their systems. Malnutrition, chronic dehydration and chemical imbalances result from this loss of essential nutrients and vital body fluids. Then the real trouble starts. Low blood potassium levels, for example, can cause heart rhythm disturbances and muscle dysfunction. Bulimics who frequently vomit to purge their systems also experience erosion of tooth enamel and may require dentures at an early age. Lying, shame, and wasting money—eating binges can get quite expensive—often accompany the eating habits they desperately try to conceal from those who love them the most. This contributes to the guilt that consumes those suffering from bulimia.

Studies have shown that most methods used to treat anorexia and bulimia are effective to some degree, but little research is available to support the benefits of one therapy over another. Psychologic approaches include behavioral therapy and modification. They have different names, but they all attempt to retrain a person to eat properly and confront the personal problems that led up to the eating disorder. Antidepressant medications have reportedly been useful additions to psychotherapy for some people, but this approach has yet to be proven over the long haul.

We've just given you a rundown on two of the most devastating eating disorders. Although they have distinct differences, the end result is the same—a severely malnourished person whose loss of judgement and distorted body image prevents information about the effects of their eating habits from getting through to them.

There are, of course, classical expressions of anorexia nervosa/bulimia. These cases are usually so pronounced and clearcut that really no questionnaire is necessary. You can pretty much point at them. But, more commonly, there are shades of grey. As is always the case, it's easier to identify black and white; more difficult to sort out the grey areas.

EAT, an acronym for the Eating Attitudes Test, is designed to help us ferret out the subtle forms of these syndromes. This quiz was developed by David E. Garner and Paul E. Garfinkel at Clark Institute of

Psychiatry at the University of Toronto. It's a quick, easy, first step to determining whether everything is alright, you have a marginal eating disorder, or whether you are literally dying to be thin. We appreciate the permission granted to us by these investigators to reproduce their questionnaire.

To each of the following questions, grade yourself:

    2 = always
    1 = sometimes
    0 = never

Do you:
1. hate the idea of gaining even a pound? ☐
2. exercise exclusively to burn calories? ☐
3. feel that your stomach should be completely flat? ☐
4. think about food most of the time? ☐
5. go on eating binges? ☐
6. feel bloated after meals? ☐
7. feel you need to diet rigorously? ☐
8. think about the fat on your body? ☐
9. feel anxious after eating high-carbohydrate foods like bread, pasta, and potatoes? ☐

10. weigh yourself more than once a day? ☐

11. avoid eating, even when you're hungry? ☐

12. take pride in being able to control your eating impulses? ☐

13. feel frightened of eating with friends and/or family? ☐

14. feel very guilty after eating? ☐

15. feel uncomfortable after eating sweets? ☐

16. feel dissatisfied with the shape of your body? ☐

17. eat or drink in secrecy? ☐

18. hate to eat the same food everyday? ☐

19. hate to have food in your stomach? ☐

20. avoid social situations that require eating? ☐

Now add up the points for all 20 questions and put your total score in the box below:

☐

Obviously, the lowest possible score is 0; the top is 40. If your final grade is 0 to 4, you're not especially preoccupied with your weight. However with a tally of 5 to 14 you're probably concerned. A grade of 15 to 24 certainly suggests weight preoccupation. Lastly, a rating of 25 to 40 may be viewed as anorexic-like thinking.

You've just completed one of the simplest tests for anorexia nervosa. As you might expect, there are many more sophisticated versions of EAT; extending into 26 and 40 questions. One of them, labeled the Eating Disorder Inventory (EDI) is now commercially available from Psychological Assessment Resources, Inc. (PAR), Post Office Box 98, Odessa, Florida 33556. For super-fast service, call 813/977-3395.

Although the EDI is a relatively new test, it can identify and differentiate subgroups with eating disorders. It distinguishes those with serious underlying mental problems from so-called "normal" dieters. It also aids in the understanding and treatment of eating disorders.

Now what to do about it?

By act, if not by word, the traditional notion is that anorexia nervosa/bulimia are really specific syndromes for which there are specific solutions. More than that, the traditional idea is that we're dealing with a fundamental psychiatric/psychologic disorder. Thus, it makes sense that the prevailing consensus is a trinity with emphasis on psychotherapy, behavior modification, and drugs (largely in the form of antidepressants). For more information, check the bibliographic material. Additionally, here are some conventional resources available. It should be underlined that the addresses and telephone numbers are correct at this writing.

The National Anorexic Aid Society, Inc. (NAAS) identifies itself as a support and educational organization for sufferers of anorexia nervosa and/or bulimia and for their families and friends. NAAS has established support groups and a national medical referral program. For more information about their membership and their quarterly newsletter, contact NAAS at 5796 Karl Road, Columbus, Ohio 43229 (telephone 614/436-1112).

Anorexia Nervosa and Related Eating Disorders, Inc. (ANRED), Post Office Box 5102, Eugene, Oregon 97405 (telephone 503/344-1144), is one of the many nonprofit organizations concerned with the overall problem of eating disorders. ANRED staff leads workshops and seminars across the United States, participates in professional conferences, works closely with Sacred Heart Hospital in Eugene, Oregon, provides a speakers' bureau, a monthly newsletter and informational packets.

The National Association of Anorexia Nervosa and Associated Disorders, Inc. (ANAD), was the first national self-help and educational society dedicated to alleviating eating disorder problems. The agency operates a national referral information center, sponsors self-help groups, develops early detection and prevention as well as educational programs, and provides information to anyone who wishes to communicate with them. They would like new chapters and self-help groups across the country. Those interested should contact the organization at Post Office Box 7, Highland Park, Illinois 60035 (telephone 312/813-3438).

The Center for the Study of Anorexia and Bulimia at the Institute for Contemporary Psychotherapy, 1 West 91st Street, New York, New York 10024 (telephone 212/595-3449), embraces five divisions, including outpatient individual and group therapy, family support programs, prevention, training and research. The prevention section distributes information and promotes the early detection of eating disorders. General informational pamphlets on anorexia and bulimia are also available upon request. There are discussion groups, workshops, and other special projects available.

Careful scrutiny suggests a more or less general agreement that the present therapy leaves much to be desired. There are several possible explanations. One may well be that the emphasis has been placed on an assumption that anorexia nervosa/bulimia is purely and simply a psychiatric/psychologic problem. It might well be that the misperceptions are not primary but actually secondary to abberations in our lifestyle. For example, the need for dietary adjustment may, in fact, be the basis for the faulty perception of weight. This can be verified, for example, by reviewing your own diet (Chapter 14). You may wish to ferret out the possible relationship of your physical activity program (Chapter 17) and/or the role of tobacco and alcohol in your own case (Chapters 15 and 16). For more and more structured analyses, check Section C: Solutions.

RESOURCES

1. Andersen, A. E.
   Practical Comprehensive Treatment of Anorexia Nervosa and Bulimia
   1985. Baltimore, The Johns Hopkins University Press.

   This book attempts a comprehensive and practical treatment program for patients with anorexia nervosa and/or bulimia. Only one method of therapy is outlined in considerable detail. This technique is derived from historical principles and approximately ten years of contact with hundreds of patients. The bases for treatment are empiric, consisting of a multifactorial concept, a team approach, and strict adherence to the historical principle of primum non nocere, which means do no harm.

2. Bruch, H.
Eating Disorders: Obesity, Anorexia Nervosa and the Person Within.
1973. New York, Basic Books, Inc.

Here's another classic which is cited by almost everyone who examines the problems of anorexia. It deals with people characterized by the abnormal amounts they eat, and they demonstrate the point by becoming conspicuous in their appearance. Anorexia nervosa, the relentless pursuit of thinness through self-starvation, even unto death, is rare indeed, certainly compared to obesity. Though anorexia nervosa deserves to be defined as a special clinical syndrome, one may also perceive it as a counterpart to obesity. In a way, it represents a caricature of what will happen when the common recommendation that reducing will make you slim, beautiful, and happy is taken too literally and carried out to the extreme.

3. Button, E. J. and Whitehouse, A.
Subclinical Anorexia Nervosa
Psychological Medicine 11: #3, 509-516, August 1981.

The Eating Attitudes Test employed in this chapter was administered to 446 female and 132 male college students and to 14 "control" subjects who met a strict diagnostic criteria for anorexia nervosa. Although none of the male students achieved high grades, a total of 28 of the female group, or 6.3 percent, scored in the "anorexic" range. These "high scorers," along with a random control group of "non-high scorers" were then interviewed. The clinical findings of anorexia nervosa were common in the high-scoring group but virtually absent in the student control group. These results appear to show that about 5% of postpubertal females display subclinical variations of anorexia nervosa. Considerable attention is relegated to a discussion of the etiology, prevention and therapy of disturbances in eating behavior.

4. Crisp, A. H.
Anorexia Nervosa: Let Me Be
1980. New York, Grune & Stratton

This classic text describes anorexia nervosa as an illness, provides a good background on the disorder, attempts to outline the mechanism and processes which underly the syndrome, and, provides a section on intervention and self-assistance. Particular attention should be paid to the self-help techniques in Chapter 13 which include a list of agencies in Great Britain and the United States which offer assistance to patients with anorexia nervosa.

5. Garfinkel, P. E. and Garner, D. M.
Anorexia Nervosa: A Multidimensional Perspective
1982. New York, Brunner/Mazel

Prepared by the Canadian originators of EAT, this text provides a detailed overview of the multidimensional nature of anorexia nervosa. The authors stress that it's the result of fashion, social expectation, familial tension, and delusional belief. The syndrome is also a product of multiple factors: starvation, which generates its own obsessions and characteristic physiologic responses, endocrinologic pathology, the difficult pattern of control-seeking, and the highly resistant disorders of self-perception. Special note should be made of Chapter 12 which deals with prognosis.

6. Garner, D. M. and Garfinkel, P. E.
The Eating Attitudes Test: An Index of the Symptoms of Anorexia Nervosa
Psychological Medicine 9: #2, 273-279, May 1979.

This report describes the development and validation of a rating scale which may be useful in evaluating a broad range of target behaviors and attitudes found in anorexia nervosa. The test is economical in terms of administration and scoring time as well as a potentially meaningful assessment and/or prognostic index. Along with the obvious advantages of EAT, there are also limitations. Self-report inventories depend heavily on the assumption that subjects will accurately describe their symptoms. This may be of particular concern with anorexia nervosa patients since they often deny they have the disorder.

7. Garner, D. M., Olmstead, M. P., Bohr, Y. and Garfinkel, P. E.
The Eating Attitudes Test: Psychometric Features and Clinical Correlates
Psychological Medicine 12: #4, 871-878, November 1982.

The Eating Attitudes Test (EAT) has been validated with anorexia nervosa patients but has also been found useful in identifying eating disturbances in others. While most of those who score highly on the EAT do not satisfy the diagnostic criteria for anorexia nervosa, personal interviews have revealed the majority do experience abnormal eating patterns which interfere with physical and mental health. Although the test may indicate the presence of symptoms common to anorexia nervosa, it would be inappropriate to assume that high scores can diagnose anorexia nervosa in nonclinical groups. And while it may indicate the presence of disturbed eating patterns, EAT does not reveal the motives for, or reasons behind, this behavior.

8. Herzog, D. B. and Copeland, P. M.
Eating Disorders
New England Journal of Medicine 313: #5, 295-303, 1 August 1985.

These investigators, from the Eating Disorders Unit, the Child Psychiatry Service and the Endocrine Unit of the Massachusetts General Hospital and the Harvard Medical School, provide a complete review of the problems of anorexia nervosa and bulimia with considerable attention directed to the natural history of these two syndromes, the physical manifestations, diagnosis, treatment, and suggestions for future directions. Although the bottom line leaves much to be desired, this report is must reading for anyone interested in a current review of eating disorders.

9. Jacobson, B.
Anorexia Nervosa and Bulimia: Two Severe Eating Disorders
1985. Toronto Public Affairs Committee Inc.

Perhaps one of the best current overviews on research and therapies that relate to these disorders. The author also delves into such areas as victims' families and psychologic development, influences of society and culture, costs and insurance coverage in the treatment of anorexia nervosa and bulimia.

10. Newman, P. A. and Halvorson, P. A.
Anorexia Nervosa and Bulimia: A Hand book for Counselors and Therapists
1983. New York, Von Nostrand Reinhold Company

This text was prepared for counselors and

therapists who are facing an ever-increasing number of young adults deeply troubled by disturbed eating habits. Developed from the counseling experiences of investigators from Moorhead State University and North Dakota State University, it offers practical suggestions that will serve in the evaluation and treatment of those with anorexia and bulimia. However, general readers concerned about their own eating habits or the eating patterns of friends or family members will also find it useful.

11. Powers, P. S. and Fernandez, R. C.
Current Treatment of Anorexia Nervosa and Bulimia
1984. New York, S. Karger.

These two faculty members from the University of South Florida brought together a group of experts to examine the overall problems of, and solutions to, anorexia nervosa and bulimia. Particular attention should be directed to an examination of the support groups listed in Chapter 17.

6

HOW'S YOUR (GOOD AND BAD) CHOLESTEROL?

We have already learned that **problems** may take different forms. To some of us, **problems** mean symptoms and/or signs. We've documented this with one of America's major complaints, fatigue, in Chapter 2. We'll come back and look at another popular problem, a mental symptom, depression, in Chapter 12.

To others with a more orthodox perspective, **problems** are viewed as discrete disease states. We underlined this point in the chapters on cancer, arthritis, and anorexia nervosa.

What has not yet been emphasized is that **problems** may take the form of biochemical aberrations such as high blood sugar, low serum calcium and elevated uric acid.

Today, there's no question but the emphasis is on measures of lipid (fat) metabolism. Until recently, principal attention was directed to total serum cholesterol and triglycerides.

- At the moment, the average total serum cholesterol in the American male is 225.
- According to the Framingham Heart Study, the man with a cholesterol level of 300 or more has triple the risk of heart attack as against someone with a cholesterol level below 175.
- For every 1 milligram percent decline in high serum cholesterol, there's a concomitant 2% reduction in coronary heart disease risk.
- According to that same Framingham study, the predictive power of serum cholesterol decreases significantly over the age of 50.

There's no question but that the popularity of cholesterol testing stems from the belief that serum cholesterol is probably the major indicator for what is now recognized as America's ultra clue of heart disease.

Before we get involved with grading our cholesterol, it might be well to clear the air and set out some of the fundamental truths and untruths about this fascinating substance.

Number one, cholesterol is a relatively simple chemical substance...a fatty alcohol!

Secondly, cholesterol is a common constituent of many foods and is an essential component of the blood. This, in itself, creates all kinds of bizarre problems and discussions. For example, it seems to logically follow that the cholesterol in the food is the cause of the cholesterol in the blood. Simply put, there is the general notion that dietary cholesterol as it were jumps into the body and becomes the blood cholesterol. The fact of the matter is, as we'll see later in this chapter, serum cholesterol and its derivitives are a function of many different lifestyle ingredients ranging from physical activity, fiber, the major foodstuffs (such as sugar and fat), vitamins and minerals.

Number three, for medical classification purposes, it's been assumed that serum cholesterol is a surefire indicator of heart disease. Actually, no biochemical parameter is characteristic of any particular disease state. Rather, biochemical testing actually brings into focus the absence or presence of the syndrome of sickness. Enlarging upon this statement, we can say with certainty that blood glucose, for example, is not the whole biochemical picture of diabetes, uric acid is not the entire story of gout, and serum cholesterol is not the only parameter of heart disease. This concept will be enlarged upon in the next chapter (p. 109)

Lastly, there are still big arguments as to what is the so-called normal serum cholesterol. History will recall, it was not too many years ago that the acceptable range was 150 to 300 mg. percent. Just a few years ago, this was changed and the experts told us that anything over 250 mg. percent was abnormal. There is increasing awareness now that possibly the upper limit should be 200 mg. percent. And to add to the confusion, even fewer researchers have given serious thought to the significance of low cholesterol.

Just for the record, we wrote a story entitled **If high cholesterol is bad...is low good?**. This report indicated clearly that both high and low cholesterol are undesirable. Further, both of these extremes correlate with a number of different problems ranging from heart disease, to cancer, and even to mental health. For more particulars, refer to this report in the Resources (p. 100).

The fact that both high and low cholesterol is not good should come as no surprise. After all, it's just as bad to be too tall as it is too short...too hot and too cold...too fat or too thin...too mad or too glad. Hence, common sense if nothing else would support the notion that both high and low total serum cholesterol reflect pathology. But more than that, there's now increasing proof that cholesterol derivatives can be more predictive than total serum cholesterol. Thus, increasing attention is being paid to high density lipoprotein cholesterol (HDL) and low density lipoprotein cholesterol (LDL).

Aside from their chemical and physical differences, what is the clinical significance?

The first point that should be made is that one can be referred to as bad cholesterol and the other good. The role bad cholesterol plays, among other things, in our lives is directly linked to cardiovascular pathosis. There's no question but coronary heart disease (CHD) follows the secret and silent process of atherosclerosis, which is the medical term for hardening of the arteries. Cholesterol aids in the buildup of plaque in the arteries of the heart. If you view your coronary arteries as drain pipes, and the plaque as something that is plugging up that pipe, you'll get a good idea of the damage it can do. When the arteries are clogged, vital blood your heart needs to function properly can't get through, and the net result is CHD. This disease is the number one killer in the United States today, according to the American Heart Association.

A massive body of scientific evidence shows that

high serum cholesterol levels, particularly when combined with tobacco consumption and high blood pressure, represent major risk factors in the development of CHD.

Our ability to differentiate between different cholesterol transport packages called lipoproteins in the blood stream has provided us with an opportunity to sharply define the cholesterol and coronary heart disease relationship. This correlation becomes even clearer when one examines the major cholesterol transport vehicle in the blood, low-density lipoprotein (LDL). The LDL that normally accounts for approximately 60% to 80% of the serum cholesterol is linked directly with coronary heart disease. Hence, this may be viewed as the **bad** cholesterol. In contrast, the high-density lipoprotein (HDL) that normally accounts for only about 15% to 25% of the serum cholesterol is inversely associated with coronary heart disease risk. In other words, high levels of HDL seem to provide some protection and therefore HDL can be viewed as **good** cholesterol.

Now, let's go to the questionnaires which, incidentally, were developed by Doctor Peter Wood, Stanford University School of Medicine, and published in Runner's World. (Reprinted by permission of Rodale's **Runner's World** Magazine. Copyright 1986.) Also, more particulars about this subject are available in the Resources (p. 107).

There are two quizzes. The first is intended to rate your blood levels of **bad** cholesterol (LDL); the other your **good** cholesterol (HDL).

First, you'll be starting with a basic LDL grade of 140. This is generally considered to be an acceptable LDL. For each factor shown in the questionnaire, choose the answer that best fits you. Enter the number given (positive, negative or zero) in the appropriate box. For example, if you're a male then insert +10; if a woman place a -1. Continue in the same way throughout. Then total your score.

starting LDL score		140

sex
male	+10	
female	-1	

family history
heart disease before 55 in immediate family	+10	
no heart disease before 55 in immediate family	0	

exercise
sedentary	+10	
some regular exercise	0	
regular aerobic exercise	-10	

weight
ideal weight or less	0	
overweight (1-29 lbs.)	+5	
overweight (30 lbs. or more)	+10	

smoking
10 cigarettes per week or more	+5	

	score	LDL
9 cigarettes per week or less	0	☐
dietary fat		
heavy fat intake	+10	☐
light fat intake	−10	☐
dietary cholesterol		
heavy intake of eggs, meats, dairy products	+20	☐
light intake of eggs, meats, dairy products	−10	☐
vegetarianism		
strict vegetarian	−10	☐
not a strict vegetarian	0	☐
TOTAL:		☐

Now to the scoring.

Give yourself an **A** if your LDL is 120 or below. Chalk up a **B** if your LDL is 121 to 199. Finally grade yourself **C** if your LDL is 200 and above.

LDL SCORE ☐

Now let's turn to the **good** cholesterol (HDL). First, you'll note that you'll be starting with a basic HDL score of 50. Once again, this is regarded as an acceptable level. For each factor shown in the questionnaire, choose the response that best fits you. Enter the number given (positive, negative, or zero) in the designated box. For example, if you're a man then insert -5 or if you are female put +5 in the box and continue in the same way throughout the questionnaire. Then total your score.

starting HDL score ☐ 50

sex
    male   -5 ☐

    female   +5 ☐

family history
    heart disease before 55
    in immediate family   -5 ☐

    no heart disease before
    55 in immediate family   0 ☐

exercise
    sedentary   -2 ☐

    some regular exercise   +10 ☐

    regular aerobic exercise   +20 ☐

weight
    ideal weight or less   0 ☐

    overweight (1-29 lbs.)   -2 ☐

    overweight (30 lbs.
    or more)   -5 ☐

smoking
    10 cigarettes per week

	score	HDL
or more	-5	☐
9 cigarettes per week or less	0	☐
dietary fat		
heavy fat intake	-5	☐
light fat intake	-2	☐
dietary cholesterol		
heavy intake of eggs, meats, dairy products	-5	☐
light intake of eggs, meats, dairy products	0	☐
vegetarianism		
strict vegetarian	+5	☐
not a strict vegetarian	0	☐
TOTAL:		☐

Assign the following values to each score. Give yourself an **A** if your HDL is 60 and above. Chalk up a **B** if your HDL is 35 to 59. Finally, grade yourself **C** if your HDL is 34 and below.

HDL SCORE ☐

Now you're ready to interpret the quiz. You're a low risk individual for heart disease if you have a score of two As or one A and one B. What this means is that your lifestyle is probably good with respect to heart disease. Hence, it's really not necessary to actually measure your HDL and LDL. View yourself as a medium risk individual if you have a score of two Bs or one A and one C. Your risk is the average for LDL or HDL. It could probably be improved by lifestyle changes. It would be wise to have your HDL and LDL measured to confirm the validity of this grading. Finally, you're a high-risk candidate if you have one score in B and one in C which predicts an increased chance of heart disease. Two scores in C suggests a very high risk. If you fall in these catagories, lifestyle changes are definitely indicated and it's clear that you should have blood measurements of HDL and LDL taken.

By the way, when you do have your cholesterol measured, keep this little tidbit of information in mind. If a technician draws blood while you're in a standing position, there's a good chance your total serum cholesterol level will measure out higher than if you're sitting or lying down. Recent studies have shown these changes can be significant, so much so in fact that they can alter the predictive potential for coronary heart disease.

And while we're at it, there are some other limitations and warnings. For example, implied if not stated in the quizzes in this chapter is that there's no upper limit to a desirable HDL and no lower nadir for LDL. We've already made mention that common sense would suggest that there must be a too high HDL and too low LDL. Pursuing the same logic, implied is the desirableness of underweight and the virtues of possible over-exercise. These are important considerations. We'll obviously not resolve them here. However, we're registering our awareness of these contradictions and hopefully they'll be considered at another time and another place.

There's no question but that orthodox medicine remains consistent. We've observed this earlier and it crops up here, namely that we're dealing with an allegedly **specific** problem for which there's pretty much a set of **specific** solutions. By act if not by word, lipid measures are considered the cardinal signals of heart disease. The specific solutions include a low fat, low cholesterol diet, weight reduction, minimum tobacco and alcohol consumption. Considerable emphasis is placed on the use of cholesterol-lowering drugs (such as cholestyramine).

In contrast, the orthomolecular community urges greater lifestyle alterations. For example, there's convincing data that serum cholesterol is similar in married couples. Additionally, the evidence shows that this is not the result of natural selection. The chemical similarities increase with time. The obvious conclusion is that this pattern must be a function of common lifestyles. This is borne out in Reference #2 on page 100. For one, it suggests significant salutary changes from a spectrum of vitamins and minerals. For example, there's now evidence of the benefits of magnesium (p. 101 and niacin (p. 105). Also, a greater effort is being placed on a search for what might be called smart agents which have the good sense, as it were, to reduce high cholesterol in high cholesterol subjects. At the same time these same agents are wise enough to elevate cholesterol in low cholesterol individuals. This is well documented in the case of vitamin C (p. 102).

Therefore you've additional options. You may examine your behavior by completing the questionnaires in Section C: Solutions and/or studying the resource material which follows.

RESOURCES

1. Cheraskin, E.
   If High Cholesterol Is Bad... Is Low Good?
   Journal of Orthomolecular Medicine 1: #3, 176-183, 1986.

   The author argues that low cholesterol levels are not necessarily good for all individuals. Citing numerous studies from several continents, positive correlations between low cholesterol and the incidence of death and numerous diverse diseases are drawn. The summary of data presented in this paper drives home the point: "How low is low" when it comes to blood cholesterol, and is it wise to continue using blanket measurements for the whole of mankind?

2. Cheraskin, E. and Ringsdorf, W. M., Jr.
   Familial Biochemical Patterns: Part I. Serum Cholesterol in the Dentist and His Wife
   Atherosclerosis 11: 247-250, March/April 1970.

   One hundred fifteen dental practitioners and their 115 wives along with 115 wives of other dentists were studied in terms of serum cholesterol levels. The evidence suggests that there's a statistically significant correlation coefficient between serum cholesterol levels only in the married couples. Within the limits of this study, the evidence indicates that this is not the result of natural selection in married couples on the basis of health status. Rather, the parallelisms become significant only with the increasing number of years together.

3. Cheraskin, E., Orenstein, N.S., and Minor, P.L.
Bio-Nutrionics: Lower Your Cholesterol in 30 Days
1986. New York, Perigee Books.

This book is intended for lay-educational purposes. It makes clear that one can significantly lower elevated serum cholesterol (as well as favorably modify other clinical and biochemical parameters) in a matter of a few days. Secondly, the obvious common denominator is that clinical and biochemical parameters which are initially above normal tend to decline toward normal; those subnormal tend to rise to near or within optimal ranges. Finally, the text underlines the fact that these changes are possible with relatively simple lifestyle modifications such as diet, vitamin/mineral supplementation, physical activity, changes in tobacco and alcohol.

4. Davis, W.H., Leary, W.P., Reyes, A.J. and Olhaberry, J.V.
Monotherapy with Magnesium Increases Abnormally Low High Density Lipoprotein Cholesterol: A Clinical Assay
Current Therapeutic Research 36: #2, 341-346, August 1984.

This investigation was undertaken to determine whether the atherogenic plasma cholesterol profile could be improved by magnesium supplementation. Sixteen adults with abnormally low HDL, significantly high LDL and normal kidney function were medicated with enteric-coated magnesium chloride as monotherapy for a period of 118 days. Total plasma cholesterol decreased, HDL rose and LDL declined. There were no undesirable effects noted. Hence, magnesium therapy should be considered as a possible option for the pharmacologic treatment of the coronary risk patient since it is very obvious that it is much safer than many of the drugs presently used.

5. Ginter, E.
Vitamin C and Plasma Lipids
New England Journal of Medicine 294: #10, 559-560, 1976.

The fundamental reason for this Letter-to-the-Editor stems from the observation that serum cholesterol levels tend to be low, possibly too low, in vegetarians. From studies done by this investigator, the conclusion is drawn that vitamin C supplementation not only is smart enough to lower cholesterol in individuals with a too high blood cholesterol (hypercholesteralemia) but also wise enough to elevate serum cholesterol in subjects with low blood cholesterol (hypocholesteralemia).

6. Hagan, R. D., Upton, S. J., Avakian, E. V., and Grundy, S.
Increases in Serum Lipid and Lipoprotein Levels with Movement from the Supine to

Standing Position in Adult Men and Women
Preventive Medicine 15, 18-27, 1986.

The effect of movement from the supine to the standing position on the magnitude of change in serum lipid and lipoprotein levels and its impact on predicting coronary heart disease was studied in 23 men and 18 women. This study, discovered posture related increases in serum lipids and lipoproteins were similar among men and women. Their results showed an increase from the supine to standing positions of 9.3 percent for total cholesterol, 9.0 percent for LDL and 10.4 percent for HDL. It's obvious that body position at time of blood withdrawal significantly influences lipid and lipoprotein levels. This can alter the predictive risk for coronary heart disease.

7. Hermann, W. J., Jr., Ward, K., and Faucett, J.
The Effect of Tocopherol on High-Density Lipoprotein Cholesterol: A Clinical Observation
American Journal of Clinical Pathology 72: #5, 848-852, November 1979.

A significant redistribution of cholesterol in lipoproteins following ingestion of large dosages of alpha tocopherol (a form of vitamin E) is documented. In subjects with low HDL, it was shown that HDL increased with vitamin E supplementation.

8. Kohls, D. J., Kies, C., and Fox, H.
Blood Serum Lipid Levels of Humans: Effect of Arginine, Lysine, and Tryptophan Supplements
Federation Proceedings 44: #5, 1498, 8 March 1985.

The amino acids arginine and tryptophan are considered to possibly lower serum cholesterol levels according to this study conducted at the University of Nebraska. Healthy subjects were first fed a control diet and then foods supplemented with one of three amino acids: arginine, lysine, or tryptophan. At the end of each two week period, fasting blood samples were drawn to test for total cholesterol and HDL. Arginine lowered total cholesterol but showed no effect on HDL. Tryptophan not only decreased total cholesterol but it also raised HDL-cholesterol. Finally, both of these effects, it should be pointed out, are considered beneficial in minimizing the risk for heart disease. Lysine supplementation exerted no effect upon serum lipids.

9. McDonagh, E. W., Rudolph, C. J., and Cheraskin, E.
Serum Cholesterol and the Aging Process
Medical Hypotheses 7: #6, 685-694, June 1981.

Two hundred and twenty-one routine patients were studied before and after approximately two months of routine therapy including EDTA treatment and general supportive care including multivitamin-mineral supplementation. The evidence indicates, within the limits of this kind of study conducted in a private practice environment, that favorable changes occurred in serum cholesterol levels suggesting a possible reversal of the aging process.

10. Odetti, P., Cheli, V., Carta, G., Maiello, M., and Vivani, G. L.
   Effect of Nicotinic Acid Associated with Retinol and Tocopherols on Plasma Lipids in Hyperlipoproteinaemic Patients.
   Pharmatherapeutica 4: #1, 21-24, 1984.

The evidence suggests that nicotinic acid lowers serum cholesterol and favorably influences the ratio of HDL to LDL ratio by increasing the HDL and lowering the LDL. The suggestion is therefore made that this fraction of the B-complex might well play a beneficial role in reducing the risk for cardiovascular disease. Unfortunately, nicotinic acid produces adverse side effects when given in dosages of 2 grams or more. This can be countered with vitamins A and E. In both groups, total cholesterol and LDL dropped significantly and HDL increased.

11. Phillipson, B. E., Rothrock, D. W., Conner, W. E., Harris, W. S., and Illingworth, D. R.
   Reduction of Plasma Lipids, Lipoproteins, and Apoproteins by Dietary Fish Oils in Patients with Hypertriglyceridemia
   New England Journal of Medicine 312: #19, 1210-1216, 9 May 1985.

Dietary fish oils, which are rich in omega-3

fatty acids, have been reported to reduce plasma lipid levels in subjects with normal blood fat concentrations. These examiners studied the effects of fish oil in 20 individuals with high triglyceride levels in their blood. The conclusion drawn is that fish oil and fish may be useful components of diets for the treatment of patients with high triglyceride levels and for the improvement in plasma lipids and their derivatives.

12. Tran, Z. V. and Weltman, A.
Differential Effects of Exercise on Serum Lipid and Lipoprotein Levels Seen with Changes in Body Weight
Journal of the American Medical Association 254: #7, 919-924, 16 August 1985.

Ninety-five studies conducted between September 1955 and October 1983 measuring changes in human serum lipid and lipoprotein levels in response to exercise training were analyzed. Changes in body weight during exercise training may confound observed serum lipid and lipoprotein level changes. Thus, data from these studies were necessarily partitioned into those where subjects gained weight, maintained body weight, or lost body weight. Results showed differential changes in blood cholesterol, triglyceride, LDL, HDL and the three body-weight categories. The results suggest that reductions in cholesterol and LDL levels were greatest when exercise training was combined with body-weight losses.

13. Wood, P. D.

The Final Word: Down with LDL!
Healthline, 8-10, February 1985.

This report includes a fascinating questionnaire which is used in this chapter to determine good and bad cholesterol. The quiz originally appeared in the March 1984 issue of Runner's World. This particular article deals with the large governmental study showing that men age 35 to 59 with high LDL can lower their heart attack risk by taking the drug cholestyramine. However, of greater significance to the public is that the study's results extend to other means of lowering LDL. The most important of these means are diet modification (lower fat content, less cholesterol, more starches), weight loss for the overweight, and regular exercise for the sedentary. There's also evidence that increasing HDL helps prevent heart disease. Exercise, weight loss, and discontinuing smoking all encourage an increase in HDL.

7

LOW BLOOD SUGAR — THE NONDISEASE!

Several points made in chapter six bear repetition. There's no question but that blood lipids, and specifically serum cholesterol and its subsets (LDL and HDL) are our most currently acceptable forecasters of heart and blood vessel disease. Secondly, there's more than common sense to suggest that both extremes (high and low cholesterol) are clinically significant (pages 91). But, most relevant here, is the fact that total cholesterol and its fractions at the present time represent the most commonly employed biochemical test in clinical medicine.

It was not always so. As a matter of fact, serum cholesterol is a johnny-come-lately on the biochemical scene.

Until just a few years ago, actually since the 1920s, the most fashionable biochemical parameter was blood sugar; more recently blood glucose. For most of us (even including many medical doctors), blood sugar and blood glucose are viewed as synonymous. This isn't true. Blood sugar equals blood glucose plus other reducing substances (like vitamin C). Hence, blood sugar is characteristically higher than blood glucose. It's stated in traditional textbooks that the difference is about 20 milligrams percent. In other words, if the blood sugar is 100, then the blood glucose is probably 80 milligrams percent. This isn't true. In point of fact, blood sugar can vary from blood glucose by 0 to as much as 70 milligrams percent. Be that as it may, blood sugar/glucose was extensively measured because the general thinking recognized the increasing incidence and prevalence of diabetes and especially maturity-onset diabetes mellitus. In those old days, it was held that about one percent of Americans had and knew they had diabetes; one percent had it and didn't know it. So, in the 1920s and 1930s the acceptable figures were that two out of every 100 run-of-the-mill Americans suffered with diabetes. Today there are even experts who hold that one out of four people in the U.S.A., during their lifetime, will have diabetes or high blood sugar indistinguishable from diabetes! There are still arguments about the scope of the high blood sugar problem.

For sure, even more confusing is the flip side—low blood sugar. It's a known historic fact that in 1949 the American Medical Association conferred its highest scientific award, the Distinguished Service Medal, on Dr. Seale Harris of Birmingham, Alabama, for research that led to the discovery of hypoglycemia. Dr. Harris was the first to observe that many patients who were not diabetic and had not been given insulin treatments appeared to go into **insulin shock**. He also noted that some patients showed the same reactions as diabetics who accidentally overdosed themselves with insulin. Could these patients be overproducing insulin in their own bodies? His suspicion was confirmed. Furthermore, he found that diet was frequently to blame.

The American Medical Association, after applauding Dr. Harris' findings more than three decades ago, did an astonishing turnabout in 1973. It labeled hypoglycemia a **nondisease**. Notwithstanding, a significant segment of the medical community has recognized the importance of what is variously labeled a disease—low blood sugar syndrome.

Common sense suggests, as we have indicated elsewhere (p. 92) that one can be too tall or too short, too fat or too thin, too mad or too glad. We've discovered in the last chapter that cholesterol can be too high or too low. Employing the same logic there's every reason to believe that, just as in the case of high blood sugar, there must be situations associated with hypoglycemia. There ought not to be an argument about that. The basis for the debate should be twofold. First, how low is low blood sugar (we'll tune in on this a bit later)? Secondly, and for now the main issue, what are the clinical ramifications of whatever low blood sugar is recognized to be?

Let's look at how far reaching this story can be. As for airline pilots, Dr. Charles R. Harper, former regional medical director for United Airlines, tested 175 pilots over the age of forty and found evidence of low-blood-sugar conditions in 44 of them...a whopping 25%! Dr. Harper suggests that airline stewardesses could contribute further to aviation safety if they stopped shuttling back and forth to the cockpit with coffee, soft drinks, and sweet rolls for the vulnerable crew.

Dr. Sam E. Roberts, professor emeritus at the University of Kansas School of Medicine, believes that marital difficulties may frequently be aggravated by unsuspected hypoglycemia. In **Exhaustion: Causes and Treatment**, he recommends that any married couple thinking of divorce should take the low-blood-sugar test if one or the other is exhausted or their dispositions are combative or violent.

Third, there's an increasing body of fact that demonstrates that unusual behavior (even of a criminal character) can be associated with low blood sugar. The writings of Alexander G. Schauss and Stephen J. Schoenthaler amply document the relationship between body chemistry and particularly hypoglycemia with bizzare and asocial behavioral patterns.

Next, and it would be well to look at the alcoholism chapter, a number of lower animal and human studies attest to the possible connection between carbohydrate metabolism and the devastations of the alcoholic syndrome.

Finally, there is the work of Dr. H. J. Roberts of West Palm Beach, Florida in the New England Journal of Medicine showing that in a group of 35 migraine sufferers given a six-hour glucose tolerance test, all 35 were diagnosed as hypoglycemic!

The frustrating point is that the clinical syndrome associated with low blood sugar is so diverse that it's difficult if not impossible to spell out a specific set of symptoms and signs. This, it should be recalled, flies in the face of traditional efforts for specificity (p. 46, 65 and 91).

And the issue is made even more confusing by the

fact that there's little agreement among the experts as to how low the blood sugar must be to be considered low. In general, some scientific releases argue that something in the neighborhood of 40 to 50 milligrams percent or less for blood glucose represents the demarcation lines. Others challenge these arbitrary numbers and recommend that the nadir depends as much if not more on the rate of decline of blood sugar rather than its absolute value. In other words, an abrupt drop in blood glucose from 180 to 80 milligrams percent, for example, may elicit more obvious clinical symptomatology than a slow decline to 50 milligrams percent. In any case, for our purposes, there are still big arguments as to the lower physiologic limits for blood glucose.

Many people first suspect the real cause of their nervous, overwrought condition after reading about low blood sugar. If suspicious that you're a smoldering undetected hypoglycemic, it's time to seek accurate verification.

A simple, self-administered questionnaire that can help you to make a presumptive diagnosis has been devised by John F. Bumpus, M.D. a Denver physician-surgeon. We wish to thank Dr. Bumpus for allowing us to use his test.

The instructions are very simple. Check only those symptoms that apply in your case. Leave blanks where answers don't apply. To indicate degrees of severity, use the following figures: 1 equals mild, 2 for moderate and 3 signifies intense.

1. abnormal craving for sweets ☐

2. afternoon headaches ☐

3. alcohol consumption ☐

4. allergies—tendency to asthma, hay fever, skin rash, etc. ☐

5. awaken after few hours' sleep—hard to get to sleep ☐

6. aware of breathing heavily ☐

7. bad dreams ☐

8. bleeding gums ☐

9. blurred vision ☐

10. brown spots or bronzing of skin ☐

11. bruise easily (black and blue spots) ☐

12. butterfly stomach, cramps ☐

13. can't decide easily ☐

14. can't start in a.m. before coffee ☐

15. can't work under pressure ☐

16. convulsions ☐

17. crave candy or coffee in afternoons ☐

18. cry easily for no reason ☐

19. depressed ☐

20. dizziness ☐

21. drink _____ cups of coffee daily ☐

22. eat when nervous ☐

23. fearful ☐

24. hallucinations ☐

25. hand tremor ☐

26. heart palpitates if meals missed or delayed ☐

27. highly emotional ☐

28. hunger between meals ☐

29. insomnia ☐

30. inward trembling ☐

31. irritable before meals ☐

32. lack energy ☐

33. magnify insignificant events ☐

34. moods of depression, blues or melancholy ☐

35. poor memory ☐

36. reduced initiative ☐

37. weakness, dizziness ☐

38. worrier, feel insecure ☐

39. chronic fatigue ☐

40. chronic nervous exhaustion ☐

41. eat often or get hunger pains or faintness ☐

42. faintness if meals delayed ☐

43. fatigue, eating relieves ☐

44. get shaky if hungry ☐

45. sleepy after meals ☐

46. sleepy during day ☐

47. symptoms come before breakfast? (answer no zero; yes with a 1) ☐

48. do you feel better after breakfast than before? (answer no zero; yes with a 1) ☐

Finished? Now add up the points you have inserted in the blanks. Put your score in the box below.

☐

Having observed thousands of these scores, Dr. Bumpus has concluded that anyone with a total grade of 25 or more should be tested further for hypoglycemia. Some symptoms are more diagnostic than others. If you answered yes to any three of questions 39 through 46, you're likely to be suffering at least some sugar intolerance.

So what do we do to help overcome low blood sugar?

We have the same two options that we've outlined in preceding chapters. For one, we can examine the low blood sugar syndrome as viewed by the conservative and traditional medical community. As we've seen, a sizable group of practitioners contend that the disease is, in fact, a nondisease. For these experts, one need do nothing. Just forget it. It's all in your head. For some of these authorities, the recommendations include standard psychotherapy with possible behavioral changes and maybe even drugs to mute the bothersome psychologic symptoms and signs.

In alternative circles, the situation is quite different. First, there's the recognition that low blood sugar, in some way, is or results in a disease. Admittedly, there are arguments about the sequence of events. Is hypoglycemia the cause of the clinical problems? Is low blood sugar simply a reflection of whatever still-to-be identified is the etiologic agent?

For sure, we're dealing with a multifactorial problem. The literature (including the resources at the end of this chapter) suggests a significant relationship between refined carbohydrate consumption to low blood sugar. This particular point is emphasized in questions 39 through 46.

Phrased simply, the reduction or better the elimination of sugar and sugar products will significantly and favorably ameliorate to some degree the low blood sugar problem in most individuals. If you want more particulars about diet and hypoglycemia check chapter 14. You might wish to take the general quiz. Parenthetic mention should be made that, in that chapter, also there's a special questionnaire intended to assess refined carbohydrate consumption.

But one should add that there are other and significant dietary contributions. For example, all things being equal, eating smaller and more frequent meals will also help solve hypoglycemia. A moderate protein and fat along with a high complex carbohydrate regime is usually beneficial. The addition of a number of vitamins (e.g. thiamine and vitamin C especially) as well as minerals (such as zinc and chromium) may also produce salutary effects.

Other nondietary factors also play a significant role. There's reasonable evidence that a sensible physical activity program along with a reduction or elimination of tobacco and alcohol can make for serious and beneficial reverberations. For a better idea of how these nonnutritional forces influence the problem, please refer to chapters 15, 16 and 17.

What can one conclude from this convoluted analysis? For one, traditional medicine at one time accepted the relatively common syndrome of hyperinsulism and its clinical expression, namely reactive hypoglycemia. Remember the story of Dr. Seale Harris? Secondly, the traditionalists have since rejected their own earlier thinking. They would contend that only rarely (and only in the case of an insulinoma, a pancreatic tumor) is there a low blood sugar disease. At best, it's their contention that we're ordinarily dealing with a relatively insignificant set of nonspecific psychologic complaints. Thirdly, in contrast, orthomolecular practitioners hold that reactive hypoglycemia is common and usually expresses itself largely in mental and emotional behavioral patterns. Next, among sophisticated investigators, there's increasing evidence that hypoglycemia in some way influences every cell, tissue, organ, and site of the body. Hence, it's not surprising that there are now reports showing the relationship of low blood sugar to a number of nonmental symptoms and signs such as dry mouth, dry socket, gingival tenderness, burning tongue and even the number of teeth (you may wish to check this out in the resources). Finally, while the cause-and-effect connections are still open to argument, there seems to be reasonable evidence that altering lifestyle by dietary and nondietary techniques can significantly modify the low blood sugar syndrome.

Additional confirmations that such is the case may be obtained from the succeeding bibliographic resources.

RESOURCES

1. Abrahamson, E. M. and Pezet, A. W.
   Body, Mind and Sugar
   1951. New York, Henry Holt and Company

   This classic textbook assembled a score of seemingly separate syndromes. The authors show common denominators in the wrecking of a train, burnout in a baseball pitcher, the seeming unexplainable suicide or homicide, and a host of other apparently bizarre mental and emotional behaviors. In short, they resolve the time-tested debate of the body-mind versus mind-body controversy. This book is about the extraordinary part that blood sugar plays in the mechanism that keeps body and mind in healthy balance.

2. Barnes, B. O.

Hope for Hypoglycemia
1978. Fort Collins, Robinson Press, Inc.

The author points out that one of the effects of sluggish liver activity is impaired carbohydrate metabolism. Additionally, in patients with poor thyroid function, the liver is unable to produce sufficient sugar during periods of stress, and hypoglycemia eventuates. Hence, the unusual contribution of this book to this chapter is the emphasis that thyroid function restores the liver to normal activity. In other words, this investigator introduces the potential element of hormonal activity into the area of carbohydrate metabolism.

3. Cheraskin, E. and Ringdorf, W. M., Jr.
Epilepsy and the Cortisone-Glucose Tolerance Test
The Journal-Lancet 88: #6, 248-250, June 1963.

The general consensus has been through studies of fasting and nonfasting blood sugar and blood glucose that there's no relationship between carbohydrate metabolism and epilepsy of the convulsive type. This experiment consists of an analysis of the cortisone-glucose tolerance test findings in 22 patients paired with respect to age and sex and including 11 epileptic and 11 nonepileptic individuals. The findings show significantly lower blood glucose levels at every temporal point except the thirty-minute determinations in the epileptic group.

4. Cheraskin, E., and Ringsdorf, W. M., Jr.
Gingival Tenderness and Carbohydrate Metabolism
American Journal of the Medical Sciences 246: #6, 727-732, December 1963.

Two hundred and ninety patients were questioned regarding the absence or presence of gingival tenderness. One hundred and twenty individuals in this group were examined by the classical glucose tolerance test, and the remaining 170 by means of the then-popular cortisone-glucose tolerance technique. It appears that there is no tie-in between gingival tenderness when one views the problem dichotomously (hyper-versus nonhyperglycemia or diabetes mellitus versus no diabetes mellitus). However, if one examines the data in a trichotomy (hyper-, normo-, and hypoglycemia), the results are different and more meaningful. In fact, there appears to be a distinct correlation between this particular symptom and carbohydrate metabolism. More accurately, gingival tenderness seems to correlate with both relative hyper- and hypoglycemia.

5. Cheraskin, E. and Ringsdorf, W. M., Jr.
Dry Mouth and Dysglycemia
Journal of the American Medical Association 229: #5, 523, 29 July 1974.

Scant attention has been given to the possible association of xerstomia (dry mouth) and overall carbohydrate metabolism (hyperglycemia, normoglycemia, and hypoglycemia). Considering these three aspects of glycemia, there appears to be a distinct correlation between xerostomia and dysglycemia, both hyperglycemia and hypoglycemia. In an age and sex paired analysis of 38 subjects, a classic three-hour glucose tolerance test was run on 19 subjects with, and 19 without, a chief complaint of dry mouth. Although there was no statistically significant difference in the mean values, the variances were highly significant at ever temporal point. These findings corroborate a dramatic disruption of blood glucose homeostasis. Here's another example of a connection between carbohydrate metabolism and a so-called mental complaint.

6. Cheraskin, E., Ringsdorf, W. M., Jr. and Brecher, A.
Psychodietetics
1974. New York, Stein and Day (hardback)
1976. New York, Bantam Books (paperback)

This book is unique by virtue of the fact that it was one of the first lay-educational expressions of the food-and-mood connection. Its relevance here stems from a number of sections. For one, there's an extensive portion of a chapter dealing with the fundamentals of hypoglycemia. Secondly, discussions are included regarding low blood sugar and alcoholism. Finally, this simple book emphasizes the possible relationships between low blood sugar and mental and emotional symptomatology.

7. Hofeldt, F. D.

Preventing Reactive Hypoglycemia: The Great Medical Dilemma
1983. St. Louis, Warren H. Green, Inc.

This book is essentially a classical analysis of the overall problem of hypoglycemia. It, however, differs from the other conventional text referred to in this section by Service (Reference #11). Doctor Hofeldt admits to a greater frequency of reactive hypoglycemia than traditionally held. However, he claims that is not as common as is recognized in alternative care systems.

8. Riordan, H. D., Cheraskin, E., Dirks, M. J., Tadayon, F.
   When are Blood Glucose Levels High (or Low) Enough to Warrant Treatment?
   In preparation

Blood glucose and Cornell Medical Index patient symptom data are reported. The results show a clear continuous and positive correlation between number of symptoms and signs and deviation from the ideal glucose score for the one to five hour postprandial time frames. A case is made for considering diabetes a treatable multidimensional disease with gradations which are evident years before the patient reaches textbook-defined biochemical and/or clinical characteristics. The ideal blood glucose range appears to be very restrictive suggesting greater correlation between both hyper- and hypoglycemia and clinical symptoms and signs.

9. Roberts H. J.
Allergy
The New England Journal of Medicine 268: #10, 562, 7 March 1963.

In an innovative investigation of migraine and so-called histamine headaches, the author reports the rarity with which an allergic explanation can be either asserted or proved and by the frequency with which recurrent hypoglycemia can provoke such headaches. In 35 out of 35 cases the classic early-morning onset of histamine headaches coincides precisely with the expected maximal decline in blood glucose concentrations in patients with functional hyperinsulinism or with recurrent hypoglycemia associated with diabetes mellitus. Furthermore, migrainous attacks can be prevented by such relatively simple measures as abstaining from sugar and sweets.

10. Ruggiero, R.
The Do's and Don'ts of Low Blood Sugar: An Everyday Guide to Hypoglycemia
1988. Hollywood, Florida, Frederick Fell Publishers, Inc.

This is an appropriate contribution because it's the story of an alleged mental patient who was subjected to the traditional psychotherapeutic regime (including even shock therapy). What's noteworthy is that the solutions to her so-called mental condition became possible only when a diagnosis of low blood sugar was made and the standard and simple orthomolecular therapy was instituted.

11. Service, J. F.
Hypoglycemic Disorders: Pathogenesis, Diagnosis, and Treatment
1983. Boston, G. K. Hall Medical Publishers

This book, the product of a number of authors and additional contributions by the senior contributor (from Mayo Clinic), provides an up-to-date and fairly traditional analysis of the overall problem of hypoglycemia. Provided is the conventional and acceptable range of blood glucose from 60 to 150 milligrams percent and the suggestion that less than 50 milligrams percent may be associated with low blood sugar. There's the admitted possibility of reactive hypoglycemia but no figures are given regarding its incidence and prevalence.

8

DON'T LET STRESS KILL YOU!

Stress is a modern metaphor, the buzzword of the 1980s. If you don't believe it just look at the incredible burgeoning of stress management courses for everybody from corporate executives to burnout babies. Who hasn't found their conversation infested with cliches of **stressful** situations, **stress-induced** problems, and **stress** syndromes?

Notwithstanding, most people are really, even if they don't know it, confused about its definition.

Simply put, stress is the result of how we deal with life events. And peeking through one of those fascinating kaleidoscopes, stress is labeled as a problem.

Actually, stress is not the problem. The problem(s) are really a series of events which are called stressors. They can be either positive (pluses) or negative (minuses). In scientific parlance, there are **eustressors** and **distressors**.

For example, Joe feels a tremendous burden when he's got too much of a workload at the office, while Sam thrives on the challenge of getting more done. In both instances, work is a stressor. However, in the former it's undesirable and in the latter it's salutary.

The negative and positive reverberations of stressors on a broad range of emotional and physical illnesses have been well-documented over the last several decades. In fact, it's abundantly clear that there's not a single cell, tissue, organ, site or system that's not significantly modified by these stressors. Experts agree this phenomenon is a predictable physiologic and psychologic response of the body to anything we perceive as challenging. The daily grind, domestic hassels, freeway traffic, the kids fighting, car trouble, and even something as seemingly insignificant as the next door neighbor's dog barking, are all stressors we all have to deal with. However, just as stressful may be an impending marriage or the pleasurableness of a high school graduation. When we encounter such situations, and more dramatic ones like death in the family, divorce, or getting a new job, our body gears up to combat or escape these stressors. This is called the **fight or flight** reaction and it triggers widespread organismal echos.

Since, in the modern world, few of life's more distressing events can be dealt with effectively by running away or fighting, the end result is frustration.

One consequence is widespread hormonal upheaval. Here's an example:

A close colleague was in a meeting one day and the chairman of her department chewed her out in front of the whole group. In a situation like this the body reacts by preparing to punch the boss or to run away. Since she couldn't do either without losing her job, she had to sit there and take it. Throughout the rest of the meeting her body became a highly charged explosive. With each tick of the clock more dynamite was added to the bomb. When the meeting was over, she stalked back to her office and stewed the rest of the day. She kept replaying that distasteful scene over and over in her mind, which in turn kept squeezing out a fresh supply of stress-related hormones.

At the end of the day, she had a headache, a stomach ache, and probably went home and raised Cain with her husband and the kids. If not, then she internalized her feelings and her body kept pumping away, producing the undesirable stress-associated hormones. It's really a vicious cycle.

Had she been able to successfully put that office confrontation in its proper place—and we'll show you ways to do that later in this chapter—those stress-hormonal juices never would have been able to do their damage, either to her body or psyche.

Stressors can also interfere with the body's natural defense mechanisms, called the immune system. When that happens a veritable Pandora's Box of physical and mental complaints is opened.

Realizing to what degree you suffer with the stress syndrome, and identifying the challenges which are causing problems, is the first step that must be instituted. The following questionnaire does just that. Incidentally, it was created by the American Medical Association and published in their book entitled **American Medical Association Family Medical Guide** (copyright 1982 by Random House, Inc.). We gratefully acknowledge permission to use it here.

You'll note there are 23 questions. Each is to be answered by a yes or no. If the response is affirmative, then place in the box the assigned number. For example, if you answer the first question yes, (has your husband or wife died within the past six months?), then you must place 20 points in the appropriate space. It's well to emphasize that these mentioned events occurred within the last six months.

1. Has your wife or husband died? (20)

2. Have you become divorced or separated from your partner? (15)

3. Has a close relative (other than husband or wife) died? (13)

4. Have you been hospitalized because of injury or illness? (11)

5. Have you married or had a reconciliation with your husband or wife after a separation? (10)

6. Have you found out you are soon to become a parent? (9)

7. Has there been a major change, whether for better or worse, in the health of a close member of your family? (9)

8. Have you lost your job or retired? (9)

9. Are you experiencing any sexual difficulties? (8)

10. Has a new member been born or married into your immediate family? (8)

11. Has a close friend died? (8)

12. Have your finances become markedly better or worse? (8)

13. Have you changed your job? (8)

14. Have any of your children moved out of the family home or started or finished school? (6)

15. Is trouble with in-laws causing tension within your family? (6)

16. Is there anyone at home or at work whom you dislike strongly? (6)

17. Do you frequently have premenstrual tension? (6)

18. Have you had an important personal success, such as a rapid promotion at work? (6)

19. Have you had jet lag (travel fatigue) at least twice? (6)

20. Has there been a major domestic upheaval, such as a move or extensive remodeling of your house (though not a change in family relationships)? (5)

21. Have you had problems at work that may be putting your job at risk? (5)

22. Have you taken on a substantial debt or mortgage? (3)

23. Have you had a minor brush with the law, such as being ticketed for a traffic violation? (2)

total

What does this all mean? Remember, this deals exclusively with events during the last six months.

The higher your overall score, the more disstressful is your life. Should your grade be **60 or more**, the pressures on you are substantial. This means that you're at a higher risk for one or more stress-related problems, as described earlier. As a general guide, a score of **under 30** suggest that you're not very likely to have a stress-associated illness or accidental injury now or in the near future.

A final word! Since the stress syndrome doesn't discriminate when it comes to age, you may wish to measure your child's challenges. For example, recent research has shown that increased life stress levels are significantly associated with drug use among adolescents. This may well turn out to be the appropriate first step in identifying a potential problem.

While modern medical literature has been paying more and more attention to adult stresses and strains, children, too, fall prey to the psychophysiologic pressures and pitfalls. And why shouldn't they? Children live in the same world, and because of age constraints and emotional immaturity often feel a helplessness that is unparalleled in adult life.

The challenges to children are not to be taken lightly. It's been linked to near epidemic episodes of adolescent suicide, and even toddlers suffering from stress (as mentioned earlier in this chapter) are being dubbed baby burnouts. Drug use among elementary school age children has increased at an alarming rate. Some investigators now estimate as many as 90 percent of all kids have experimented with alcohol, marijuana, or other drugs before they reach the tender age of 14. More details are available in Chapter 16.

Is your child under stress? The following questionnaire developed by Eugene Raudsepp, Ph.D., and printed in the July 1986 issue of Harper's Bazaar is geared for parents of children between the ages of four and twelve. It will give you a clue as to how much pressure your child is feeling right now and how well he or she is handling it. Permission to use this form has been given by the inventor.

Answer each question by checking off the item that most accurately describes the situation as it actually is, not how you'd like it to be. You must be brutally honest to obtain valid results on this quiz. Respond to each question with A for often, B for sometimes, C for seldom and D for never. You'll note each box has an assigned value above it. For example, if your answer to question 1 is sometimes (which is B), then place a 4 in the appropriate box.

1. How often does your child (he or she is implied throughout) experience any of these symptoms: headaches, stomach pains or other digestive problems, tight muscles, shortness of breath, difficulty swallowing, cold hands or feet, sores in mouth, sweaty palms or increased perspiration?

    A(8)　B(4)　C(1)　D(0)

2. How often does he exhibit these symptoms: trembling or shaking, stuttering, shaky voice, nervous tics, frowning or wrinkling of forehead, grinding or clenching teeth, skin rashes, colds, low-grade infections, allergies, sleeping difficulties, severe fatigue?

    A(8)　B(4)　C(1)　D(0)

3. How often is he restless, irritable and in a low mood?

    A(7)　B(3)　C(1)　D(0)

4. Does he feel too many demands are made on him and that there is not enough time for play?

    A(5)　B(2)　C(0)　D(0)

5. Does he ever seem anxious or apprehensive even though he doesn't know what has caused it?

    A(5)　B(2)　C(1)　D(0)

6. Does he ever act withdrawn, listless or apathetic?

   A(6) B(3) C(1) D(0)

7. Does he have difficulty expressing how he feels about situations or people?

   A(4) B(2) C(0) D(0)

8. Does he ever act sullen or defiantly aggressive?

   A(4) B(2) C(0) D(0)

9. Does he have any recurring nightmares?

   A(5) B(2) C(1) D(0)

10. Does he have crying spells?

    A(4) B(2) C(0) D(0)

11. How often does he quarrel with you, your spouse or with siblings?

    A(4) B(2) C(1) D(0)

12. Is he concerned about his appearance (weight, height, etc.); does he feel unattractive?

    A(5) B(3) C(0) D(0)

13. Does he tend to overeat, especially sweets?

    A(4) B(2) C(0) D(0)

14. Is he exposed to family arguments or quarrels?

    A(5) B(2) C(0) D(0)

15. Is he ever punished for "not telling the truth?"

    A(4) B(2) C(0) D(0)

16. Does he ever feel deprived of the freedom and privileges other children his age enjoy?

    A(4) B(2) C(0) D(0)

17. Does he ever feel envy or resentment that someone has something he does not?

    A(4) B(2) C(0) D(0)

18. Are there tight restraints on what he may or may not do?

    A(4) B(2) C(1) D(3)

19. Is he pressured to do well in school?

    A(4) B(2) C(3) D(4)

20. Does he have any problems concentrating on schoolwork?

    A(5) B(3) C(1) D(0)

21. How often is he tardy or absent from school?

    A(5) B(2) C(0) D(0)

22. Does he tend to fall behind with schoolwork?

    A(5) B(2) C(0) D(0)

23. Is he satisfied with his accomplishments in school?

    A(0) B(0) C(3) D(5)

24. Does he ever fail to understand or do homework assignments?

    A(3) B(1) C(0) D(0)

25. Does he tend to worry about what his teachers think of him?

    A(4) B(2) C(0) D(0)

26. Does he ever complain of boredom with school?

    A(5) B(3) C(1) D(0)

27. Does he ever feel excluded from peers, classmates or friends?

    A(5) B(3) C(0) D(0)

          yes   no

28. Of late, do you find your child more short-tempered and argumentative than usual?   5   0

29. Does he feel he can live up to your and/or your spouse's ex-

		yes	no
	pectations?	0	4
30.	Does he feel you and/or your spouse understand his problems and are supportive?	0	5
31.	Does he have brothers or sisters who are overly competitive with him?	3	0
32.	Are both you and your spouse working?	4	0
33.	Does he feel afraid for no reason at all?	4	0
34.	Does he have trouble with any schoolmates or playmates?	3	0
35.	Is he as popular with other children as he would like to be?	0	3
36.	Have his school grades taken a sudden drop of late?	4	0
37.	Is he easily fatigued when he spends even a little time studying?	5	0
38.	Has he had any behavior problems in school?	4	0
39.	Does he have trouble with any teachers?	4	0

		yes	no
40.	Has he lately taken on any extra activities or lessons he doesn't enjoy?	5	0

During the past six months, has your child experienced any of the following:

		yes	no
41.	Move to a new community?	3	0
42.	Change to a new school, class room or teacher?	3	0
43.	Change of friends (new ones, loss of old ones)?	3	0
44.	Change in the amount of TV viewing?	3	0
45.	Disappointment with a friend?	4	0
46.	Loss of a pet?	5	0
47.	Change in appetite?	4	0
48.	Loss of interest in playing with other children?	5	0
49.	Change in number of fights with siblings?	3	0
50.	Change in sleeping habits (staying up late, giving up nap, etc.)?	4	0

		yes	no
51.	Beginning new activities (sports, hobbies, music lessons, Brownies, etc.)?	5	0
52.	Witnessing delinquency, vandalism in school?	5	0
53.	Suspension or expulsion from school?	6	0
54.	Theft or loss of possessions?	5	0
55.	Personal injury or illness?	8	0
56.	Death of family member?	12	0
57.	Poor health of family member?	7	0
58.	Divorce of parents or marital separation?	9	0
59.	Birth of a new baby?	6	0
60.	Mother going to work or stopping work?	5	0

total score ☐

A grade in the 190 to 280 range shows your child is under a very high level of stress. His or her problems definitely outnumber pleasures in life. Refer to the major sources of stress as you perceive them from the test questions. You must do everything possible to eliminate unfavorable stressors in your child's life. Communication and reassurance is absolutely necessary to resolving those situations that are causing undue pressure on the child. And finally, if problems persist, don't hesitate to seek professional counsel.

Scores in the 118 to 189 spread indicate your child is either experiencing average environmental challenges or handling it quite well. Nonetheless, there's always room for improvement, so refer to the questionnaire and try to help eliminate those obvious stressors when possible.

If the number is between 3 to 117, your child's stress level is low, and he or she probably handles difficulties well. Although there may be normal minor worries, the youngster is not weighted down with problems.

There are many solutions to the **stress** problem. Some have been cited such as seeking professional help. Others can be identified with other questionnaires listed in the Solution Section of this monograph. But for the moment, here are some dos and don'ts:

Do challenge stressful thinking: As in the example of the co-worker who was chewed out by the boss, avoid reprocessing stressful thoughts over and over again. Address them, resolve them, then get on about the business of living. The anger they cause will only increase the production of unfavorable hormones.

Do be assertive: Learning to express your feelings, without aggression, is a must when it comes to managing noxious challenges. Remember, your willingness to disclose feelings could make an enormous difference in your stress response.

Do learn to slow down: The constant need to do more in less time leads many people to experience enormous amounts of frustration. It may make for some temporary accomplishments, but the end result is tantamount to swimming upstream, which in turn creates feelings of aggressiveness, hostility and excessive competition.

Do monitor your feelings: It's important to seriously analyze your feelings on a daily basis. Be honest with yourself and realize that how you perceive a particular stressor is what causes damage to your emotions and body, not the stressor in and of itself.

Don't neglect diet and exercise: There's no doubt about a food-mood connection in terms of how we deal with stressors. The same holds true for physical activity and sleep periods. Without offering your body and mind the benefit of optimal diet, exercise and sleep, the hormonal balance is greatly disrupted, allowing stressors to do their damage. If you'd like to better assess these lifestyle factors, this would be a good time to check the questionnaires in Chapters 14 (diet) and 17 (exercise). Also, review the reference **Psychodietetics** in the resources section for additional guidance.

Don't sharply increase or decrease lifestyle patterns: All changes should be made slowly and stimulating activities eased into. After all, change is a major stressor, even those that are ultimately beneficial to body and mind. Remember, the marathon runner always warms up before tackling a race. Your body, and emotions, need the same warmup period before you start something new, or begin to cut down on something you've been doing.

Don't overindulge: Exaggerating any behavior disrupts the body's natural rhythm. Moderation is a vital element in controlling distressors. Excessive amounts of alcohol, for example, can greatly disrupt the immune system and negatively affect your ability to deal with stressful situations. Obviously, the same holds true for tobacco. Questionnaires are provided for you to assess these habits in the section on solutions.

Don't expect too much from yourself: Realize that you're only human. Everyone makes mistakes and brutalizing yourself over hitting one foul ball will only make life miserable. Learning how to forgive yourself is essential in turning a negative stressor into a eustressor.

Finally, additional support may be possible by checking the succeeding Resource references.

RESOURCES

1. Bruns, C., and Geist, C. S.
   Stressful Life Events and Drug Use Among Adolescents
   Journal of Human Stress 10: #3, 135-139, Fall 1984.

   The hypothesis that increased amounts of stress during and/or prior to adolescence is associated with elevated drug use or abuse is examined. The authors conclude that increased life stress levels are significantly associated with elevated drug use. These investigators learned that stressors are cumulative and include both good and bad events. They state that getting all As on one's report card adds to stress levels, just as getting all Fs does. The researchers also learned that drug use starts, for the most part, at the junior high school age or below, and that the use of cigarettes is the entry level into the whole drug scene.

2. Cheraskin, E., Ringsdorf, W. M., Jr., and Brecher, A.
Psychodietetics
1974. New York, Stein and Day (hardback)
1976. New York, Bantam Books (paperback)

This book, written for lay educational purposes is designed especially to identify the food-and-mood connection. It's relevance here is that it includes an interesting stress questionnaire developed by Doctor Thomas Holmes (professor of psychiatry at the University of Washington), and Doctor Richard H. Rahe (of the United States Navy Medical Neuropsychiatric Unit in San Diego). Parenthetic mention should be made that the Holmes/Rahe questionnaire has served, with modifications, as a prototype for many so-called stress questionnaires.

3. Humphrey, J. H. and Humphrey, J. N.
Stress in Childhood
Selye, H.
Selye's Guide to Stress Research, Volume 3
1983. New York, Von Nostrand Reinhold Company, Incorporated, pp 136-168.

    This particular chapter in Selye's guide deals exclusively with stress and children. It includes keen insights into the characteristics of childhood emotionality; emotional arousals and reactions; guidelines for emotional development of children; factors which induce stressful challenges in children; home and school conditions which can generate stressors, and teacher behavior which can induce tensions in children. Of particular importance is a subsection which deals with child stressor reduction techniques, and principles to apply in helping children deal with the stress syndrome.

4.   Novaco, R. W.
Anger Control: The Development and Evaluation of an Experimental Treatment. 1975. Lexington, Lexington Books.

    The author, a professor in the Department of Social Ecology at the University of California at Irvine, has developed a short and interesting anger questionnaire which provides a so-called irritability quotient (IQ). This volume, according to the author, represents the first attempt to develop therapeutic methods for persons with chronic anger control problems and to evaluate the clinical procedures in a controlled experimental design.

5.   Pesznecker, B. L. and McNeil, J.
Relationship Among Health Habits, Social Assets, Psychologic Well-Being, Life Change and Alterations in Health Status

Nursing Research 24: #6, 442-447, November/December 1975.

A questionnaire was mailed to residents of Renton, Washington, to examine variables which may temper life change and enable individuals to withstand high degrees of life change without developing illness. Five hundred forty eight residents responded. Major variables in the questionnaire were health habits, social assets, psychologic well-being, and life change. Alterations in health status was the dependent variable. Results indicated that as life changes increased, the risk of becoming ill also increased.

6. Rahe, R. H.
Subjects' Recent Life Changes and Their Near-Future Illness Reports
Annals of Clinical Research 4: #5, 250-265, 1972.

Man's constitutional endowment is of major importance in his resistance and vulnerability to many disease states, and such genetic and acquired traits operate over his entire life span. Life change events, however, are temporary in their occurances and in their influence upon a person's life. Examples of life changes include the death of a spouse, divorce, incarceration, change in residence, loss of a job and major changes in financial status. Life Change Units (LCU) are numerical values assigned to various life changes. As the LCU increases in a person's life, more illnesses are reported. A study of 50 U. S. Navy and Marine Corp subjects has borne this out.

7. Rahe, C. R. H. and Arthur, R. J.
   Life Change and Illness Studies: Past History and Future Directions
   Journal of Human Stress 4: #1, 3-15, March 1978.

   The number and diversity of life changes and illness studies to date firmly establish a significant relationship between a person's recent life change experience and subsequent development and reporting of major and minor illnesses, and death. Psychosocial events are transduced in the brain into physiologic events which activate the neuroendocrine axis and other systems, such as autonomic control mechanisms.

8. Russeck, H. and Russeck, L.
   Is Emotional Stress an Etiologic Factor in Coronary Heart Disease?
   Psychosomatics 17: #2, 63-67, Second Quarter, 1976.

   For years there has been a strong clinical impression that emotional stress and personality type should be considered an important risk factor in coronary heart disease. Man has been on this planet for over three million years. He has been in factories for only 300 years. Since adaptation to changing environment generally takes hundreds of thousands of years, it's to be expected that modern man is currently being exposed to a continuing evolutionary process of natural selection to determine who shall survive. Coronary heart disease may be one means through which such selection is being accomplished.

9. Selye, H.
   Selye's Guide to Stress Research, Volume 2
   1983. New York, Van Nostrand Reinhold Company, Incorporated.

   Long regarded as the world's foremost authority on stress, this text offers an excellent overview on all aspects of the stress reaction. Dr. Selye has completed a volume which emphasizes the theoretical aspects of the stress syndrome and its many applications. Also presented are analyses of many psychosomatic implications of stress, including a discussion of hypertension and cardiovascular diseases. Contributors to the text examine stress tests; the methodologic difficulties in carrying out research in sports stress; the relation of the stress response to adaptive behavior. Additionally, there's interesting information regarding job stress, police officers, and much more.

10. Tache, J., Selye, H. and Day, S. B.
    Cancer, Stress and Death
    1979. New York, Plenum Medical Book Company.

    The stress syndrome as a factor in cancer and death is carefully explored by a diverse group of researchers. This excellent book pools information from many sources to examine the relationship between stressors in cancer and in death. The text is a valuable resource for anyone wishing an in-depth view of the multidimensional aspects of stress, cancer and death.

9

WHAT'S YOUR FINANCIAL STATE OF HEALTH?

No argument...
Money is somehow tied to health and happiness. No question, money can't do everything. For one, it won't buy poverty! On a more serious note, however, the evidence is in that poor people die younger; and before they pass away they have lots more medical problems.

True, money can't buy happiness, but try living on the edge day after day, year after year, and it'll definitely detract from one's quality of life. After all, a lack of appropriate funds to meet those needs that keep body and soul together is a negative stressor (a subject discussed in some depth in the last chapter). And so, it seems logical now to examine the woes of the wallet!

Common sense suggests that if money problems remain a constant companion, health will ultimately be affected.

Who has money problems?

First, there's a significant segment of the public that is poor by virtue of the fact that money is just not available. There are literally millions of babies and children who live under poverty conditions. Millions of elderly people have pensions that just don't stretch far enough to cover basic needs.

These poor souls (and it's variously estimated that there are somewhere between 30 and 50 million) have a problem which requires an immediate solution. The issue centers about a paradox, namely that, on the one hand, there's a literal abundance if not overabundance of food and services. On the other hand, there are segments of the population that are underfed, underclothed, and without shelter. These issues need attention. However, we're not going to solve them here. We shall have to leave this to the politicians, economists, industrialists, and all of those others who dictate the operation of the capitalists system.

According to financial experts, a lack of funds isn't what's generating all the hair-pulling days and sleepless nights. The bottom line is millions of people just don't properly manage what they do have—no matter how little (or how much) it is. Consequently, they fall deeper and deeper into debt, practicing reality avoidance, and often falling back on that all too familiar cliche "oh well, I'll take care of it next payday." When they finally do emerge from the delusion, bill collectors are already knocking at the door, late payment statements are piling up in the mailbox, and an enormous amount of tension has made itself at home in the body and the psyche. This problem isn't confined to a particular economic group. On the one hand, who hasn't noticed a lean-to shack with a television antenna poking out of the roof and a spanking new Cadillac sitting out front. On the other hand this dilemma affects even the yuppies. So what do you do about it?

There are ways to avoid the trap and pull yourself out of trouble, but like most conditions this book addresses, you have to recognize the danger signals first.

The following questionnaire is a quick first step to determining whether you're heading for financial disaster. Developed by the American Bankers Association, it identifies areas that those with financial problems have in common. (Reprinted with permission from the American Bankers Association. All rights reserved.)

Answer the following questions honestly by checking the appropriate box. Examine your score. Next, check the resources section for the literature that will help you on the road to regaining the happiness and peace of mind that comes from doing something about one of this country's favorite pastimes—poor money management.

                                            yes   no

1. Do you use credit today to buy many of the things you bought last year with cash?

2. Have you taken out loans to consolidate your debts or asked for extensions on ex-

	yes	no

isting loans to reduce monthly payments? ☐ ☐

3. Does your checkbook balance get lower by the month while your standard of living stays the same? ☐ ☐

4. Instead of paying most bills in full each month, as you did in the past, are you now paying only the minimum amount due on your charge accounts? ☐ ☐

5. Have you begun to receive repeated notices of overdue bills from your creditors? ☐ ☐

6. Have you been drawing on savings to pay regular bills that you used to pay out of your monthly paycheck? ☐ ☐

7. You've borrowed before on your life insurance policy but this time, are the chances of paying it back more remote? ☐ ☐

8. Do you now depend on extra income, such as overtime and dividends, to get you through to the end of the month? ☐ ☐

9. Do you use your checking

account "overdraft" to pay
regular monthly bills? ☐ ☐

10. Are you juggling your rent or mortgage money to pay other creditors? ☐ ☐

total ☐ ☐

If you answered yes to two of these questions, it's time to take a close look at your budget. With three affirmative replies, you may be headed for difficulty. And if five or more of these questions apply to you, you're definitely in trouble. But don't panic. According to the American Banking Association, the most important step you can take at this time is to explain your situation to your lenders.

This sounds simple, and it is. But many people feel it's a sign of personal failure when they see themselves getting into financial trouble and they make the unfortunate mistake of avoiding their lenders.

Regardless of how you scored on the questionnaire, budgeting makes good common cents (sic). The following budget planner, complete with rules and formulas for converting dollar amounts into monthly increments, is provided to help make that important first step towards financial freedom.

Some people are paid daily, others weekly or every two weeks or monthly. To simplify the calculations, an example is provided. To make matters easier, express to the nearest whole dollar amount.

Rules for converting to monthly amounts:
If your wages   Adjust as shown below:
are paid per:

day	$ amount x 365 ÷ 12
week	$ amount x 52 ÷ 12
every two weeks	$ amount x 26 ÷ 12
twice a month	$ amount x 2
irregular	work out an estimate for the year and divide by 12

(For example, should your salary be $100.00 per week, you'd multiply $100 times 52 and divide that number by 12; i.e. $100 x 52 = $5,200.00 ÷ 12 = $433.00 which represents your approximate monthly income.)

Now let's make a monthly budget planner.

Listed below are the common income and expense categories for most American households. Review each item and write down the appropriate amount for your own situation.

income:

	Column 1 ($ per pay period)	Column 2 ($ per month)	Column 3 (Budget $ per month)
take home pay			
commissions, bonuses, tips			
interest, dividends (include stock and money market mutual funds)			
real estate income			
social security, pensions			
other			
total income			

expenses:

	Column 1 ($ per pay period)	Column 2 ($ per month)	Column 3 (Budget $ per month)
Savings:			
investments			
long term savings			
short term savings			
emergency fund			
other			

subtotal: savings per month ☐

Fixed expenses:

mortgage or rent			
property taxes			
income, local taxes			
insurance:			
life			
auto			
health			
homeowners/renters			
Utilities (electricity, water, etc.)			
housing maintenance and operation			

	Column 1 ($ per pay period)	Column 2 ($ per month)	Column 3 (Budget $ per month)
bank loans			
car payments			
other debts (list)			
child care/education			

subtotal: Fixed expenses per month ☐

Flexible expenses:

food			
clothing			
medical/dental			
telephone			
transportation (gas, car repair, bus fares, etc.)			
credit cards			
home furnishings, equipment			
dry cleaning/laundry			
donations, club dues, church			
vacation money			
Christmas gifts/other gifts			

	Column 1 ($ per pay period)	Column 2 ($ per month)	Column 3 (Budget $ per month)
personal items/miscellaneous	☐	☐	☐
other	☐	☐	☐

subtotal: Flexible expenses per month ☐

To determine your total expenditures each month, add the following:

Savings per month ☐

Fixed expenses per month ☐

Flexible monthly expenses ☐

total monthly expenditures ☐

Let's now see how well you did. Put in Box A below your income. Place your expenditures in Box B. Subtract B from A to determine your financial status.

A ☐ − B ☐ = C ☐

Income   Expenditures   Difference

If, after completing your monthly budget planner, you find that your income exceeds your expenses, you should consider adding those additional dollars to your savings or investing the money. But if your expenses surpass your income, this planner will help you to examine each item carefully to ascertain where you can reduce your spending. Should you find it impossible to make your budget balance, you may wish to see a financial counselor to avoid getting too deeply in debt.

As an additional tool, try completing the shopaholic questionnaire devised by Carla Perez, M.D., which was published in the April 1987 issue of Prevention Magazine. We thank her for granting us permission to reproduce it.

Try it and see if it doesn't help explain some of your problems.

		yes	no
1.	Is shopping your major form of activity?		
2.	Do you buy new clothes that sit in the closet for weeks or even months before you wear them?		
3.	Do you spend more than 20 percent of your take-home pay to cover your loans and credit cards?		
4.	Do you ever pay one line of credit with another?		
5.	Do you pay only the minimum balance on your charge accounts each month?		
6.	Do you ever hide your purchases in the car or lie about them so your spouse doesn't know you were shopping?		
7.	Do you ever lie about how

	yes	no

much something cost so your spouse or friends think you were just after a bargain? ☐ ☐

8. Do you buy something just because it's on sale even though you have no use for it? ☐ ☐

9. When out with friends for dinner, do you offer to put the check on your credit card so you can collect the cash? ☐ ☐

10. Do you feel nervous and guilty after a shopping spree? ☐ ☐

11. Is your paycheck often gone on Tuesday when the next payday isn't until Friday? ☐ ☐

12. Do you borrow money from friends, even though you know you'll have a hard time paying it back? ☐ ☐

13. Do you frequently have to charge small purchases, such as toiletry items and groceries, because you don't have enough cash in your pocket? ☐ ☐

14. Do you think others would be horrified if they knew how much money you spent? ☐ ☐

	yes	no
15. Do you often feel hopeless and depressed after spending money?	☐	☐
total	☐	☐

Now place in the box below the total number of yeses.

☐

If you answered yes to five or more of these questions, the experts say you have a spending problem and should seek professional help. Also, you may wish to refer to the resources which follow.

There's no argument but that mismanagement is a big factor in our financial health. There's also no question but that viewing the problem as we've just done may be the entire solution but, it's also clear that filling out the questionnaires in this chapter will not provide the needed direction for lots of people.

For example, it's obvious that one possible solution is to increase one's income. Lots of folks do this with second jobs, moonlighting, and similar techniques. The impulse is to conclude that those who do not take on these extracurricular activities do so because of lack of will-power or interest. This isn't always the case. For example, studies have shown (p. 30) that one can improve productivity by simply adding small amounts of an iron supplement in people who suffer unknowingly with subclinical anemia. Hence, it might be in order to increase one's income but by techniques usually not alluded to in traditional financial texts. If you're curious to know the effectiveness of this avenue of adding income based on energy levels (see chapter 2), and/or you might wish to check your own eating habits by filling out the appropriate questionnaires in Chapter 14.

On the other hand, one of the solutions to financial ill-health is to reduce expenditures. As but one example, it should be pointed out that tobacco and alcohol are expensive hobbies. You might not realize how costly they are. To acquire this information, we'd suggest that you complete the quizzes in those respective chapters (15 and 16).

There's another way of looking at tobacco and alcohol. On balance, they are negative lifestyle habits. This is simply another way of saying that, as minuses, they discourage health and invite illness. The reduction or elimination of these and other noxious habits may reduce medicodental expenditures. This is but another way of pointing out that one can improve the financial discrepancy by reducing expenditures.

In this connection, it's noteworthy that the same lifestyle pluses and minuses discussed in earlier chapters in this section obtain here. You may wish to review them.

RESOURCES

1. Blue, R. and Blue, J.
   Money Matters for Parents and Their Kids
   1988. Nashville, Thomas Nelson Publishers

   The authors remind us of the devastating fact that four out of five Americans owe more than they own! With this in mind, this book focuses on four skills that children need to know in order to become financially mature (1) budgeting, (2) purchasing, (3) decision making, and (4) goal setting. These abilities are all founded in Biblical principles, because "the truth of financial maturation is also the basis for spiritual maturity."

2. Burkett, L.
An$wers to Your Family's Financial Que$tions
1987. Pomona, Focus on the Family.

This book utilizes a question-and-answer format to respond to Christian families' typical fiscal concerns. Divided into practical sections, the book serves as a ready reference for the family. These topics are based on questions received by the author from his radio program, financial seminars and/or books. Mr. Burkett explains not only how to handle finances but also how Scripture applies to this important area of your life.

3. Editors
How to Live on Your Income
1970. New York, Reader's Digest Association, Inc.

This is a truly comprehensive, authoritative and thoroughly practical guidebook that will show you how to solve your everyday money problems in ways you never thought possible. It covers the whole range of family finance—from buying meat for tomorrow night's dinner to financing four years of college for your son or daughter. This book will provide you with the help you need in just about every area where money is important.

4. German, D. and German, J.
   Money A to Z: A Consumer's Guide to the Language of Personal Finance.
   1984. New York, Facts on File Publications.

   Are you baffled by financial jibberish that keep springing up in conversations with people who know how to talk money? This book is the answer. It's loaded (1,400 entries) with clear, understandable definitions of financial terms. The authors also give advice on how to make the definitions work for you and discuss a broad range of subjects from bank accounts to tax savings.

5. Knight, S. and Squires, R.
   Financial Planning
   1983. Washington, D. C., American Bankers Association.

   This booklet is an excellent starting place for anyone wishing to put their financial affairs in order. It's an authoritative, easy-to-understand guide offered by the American Bankers Association. It tells you how to get started with a financial plan, how to determine your net worth, how to buy insurance, and good solid advice on basic money matters. Check lists, including one itemizing important documents that affect your finances, and a net worth planner are included.

The questionnaire in this book is the one we have cited.

6. Miller, T. J.
Make Your Money Grow: Smart Steps to Success in the Exciting Years Ahead.
1984. Washington, D. C., The Kiplinger Washington Editors, Inc.

The staff of Changing Times Magazine has packed a wealth of information into this 378 page book. Clearly written for the man-on-the-street, it shows you how to take charge of your money, use credit wisely, and where you should take your financial business. It also examines insurance options, tax shelters you can use, and fine points in buying, selling and renting a home. Many other topics are discussed in detail and a budget format for the 1980's is included.

7. Porter, S.
Love and Money
1983. New York, William Morrow and Company, Inc.

Sylvia Porter has put together a unique book that delves into the heretofore forbidden world of love and money. As she puts it, "if you're romantically involved, you're financially involved. Love and money may be the most vital parts of your life, and they are more closely intertwined than you may think." Ms. Porter speaks openly on the necessity of communication in avoiding problems in a relationship that may arise out of financial concerns. Other topics include prenuptial agreements, cohabitation agreements, checking accounts, managing money, separation agreements, divorce, budgeting, and credit. The author uses money case histories and profiles to show how love and money interact in everyone's life.

8. Sloane, L.
The New York Times Book of Personal Finance
1985. New York, Times Books.

This well-written, highly informative book by the financial columnist for the New York Times should be required reading for anyone facing financial difficulties. Mr. Sloane tells you everything you need to know about the financial decisions everyone faces at one time or another. Sound advice on credit, taxes, insurance, mortgages, investments, retirement plans and wills, is included.

9. Sprinkel, B. W. and Genetski, R. J.
Winning with Money: A Guide for your Future.
1977. Homewood, Dow Jones-Irwin.

This is not light reading, but it reads well. The authors, who are both economists and bankers, have put together a practical guide to the major economic issues and how they affect us all. (Incidentally, Mr. Sprinkel has been President Reagan's Economic Adviser.) They discuss the implications of government policies and their impact on your finances. If you want to know the mechanics of money, including the role of the Treasury and the Federal Reserve, this book is the ticket. A section on policies for prudent, and aggressive, investors is included.

10

HOW'S YOUR WORKPLACE HEALTH?

A sociologist recently asked 750 working people in Alameda County, California, to make a hypothetical choice between a two percent pay raise or a two percent reduction in worktime. Eighty-five percent took the time. When he elevated the ante to a 10 percent raise versus a 10 percent cut in worktime, three in five took the money.

The point of the story is that there's a real connection between money (the subject of the last chapter) and work (the immediate theme).

From board rooms to mail rooms, typing pools to

steel mills, health in the workplace is increasingly becoming a hot topic with bosses and workers alike.

It's about time!

Consider this. The average person spends about eight hours a day on the job. Aside from sleep, most of us are in the office, factory or some other work related environment the bulk of our waking hours. Given that fact, it should come as no surprise that your workplace **personality** could significantly modify your **health and happiness**.

So hear this:
- The average American man works 21.1 years of his life
- By about 1990, the average employee may be down to a 4-day workweek.
- In an ordinary year, 1 person in 6 changes jobs.

How do all of the above add to worksite woes?

Through the Occupational Safety and Health Administration (OSHA), work environments that pose inherent hazards, like heavy industry, chemical plants, and coal mines, undergo strict federal inspections periodically to check for dangers. But what about the more subtle factors at the office that can most adversely affect your health?

For example, you're struggling to kick the nicotine habit for the umpteenth time and a gal at the next desk lights up. As the smoke goes wafting through the air to your nostrils, you find yourself bumming just one last cigarette. On the other hand, perhaps you don't even use tobacco but find yourself one of millions who are categorized as passive smokers. They don't light up but suffer some of the same health consequences smokers eventually have to come to grips with. Of course, some companies now have designated smoking areas, but they are still few and far between.

Take another scene. Just yesterday you vowed to trim off that excess 20 pounds. Today you **had** to at least nibble at the calorie laden business luncheon, not to mention keeping up with the boss' three martini habit.

And how many days do you find yourself trying to talk on the phone but office noise is making it increasingly difficult to carry on a conversation.

And there's even more. A poll taken by USA Today summarizes many other contributing problems. Sixty-four percent of the people claim they just don't like their job. One-half tell us there's poor communication. Forty-six percent think that understaffing is a big issue. Finally, one-third indicate poor supervision is a cardinal concern.

All of these items and more highlight the point that most offices—and other work environments—pose problems. You see, the attitudes, habits and tastes of people you work with can make it very difficult to lead a healthy life. You may have been living with these problems so long you're not even aware of them.

The following questionnaire, developed by H. Jayne Vogan, an associate professor of counselor education, a stress management consultant and private psychotherapist, was printed in the 16 June 1987 issue of USA Today. And by the way, we thank Doctor Vogan for allowing us to cite this interesting questionnaire.

This test was designed to help identify on-the-job challenges. Take it and see for yourself if your tension level is normal, beginning to be a problem or dangerous. Answer each statement by placing the following assigned value in the appropriate box.

seldom true = 1
sometimes true = 2
mostly true = 3

1. Even over minor problems, I lose my temper and do embarassing things like yell or kick a garbage can.

2. I hear every piece of information or question as criticism of my work.

3. If someone criticizes my work, I take it as a personal attack.

4. My emotions seem flat whether I'm told good news or bad news about my performance.

5. Sunday nights are the worst time of the week.

6. To avoid going to work, I'd even call in sick when I'm feeling fine.

7. I feel powerless to lighten my work load or schedule, even though I've always got far too much to do.

8. I respond irritably to any request from co-workers.

9. On the job and off, I get highly emotional over minor accidents, like typos, spilt coffee.

10. I tell people about sports or hobbies

that I'd like to do, but say I never have time because of the hours I spend at work.

11. I work overtime consistently, yet never feel caught up.

12. My health is running down; I often have headaches, backaches, stomachaches.

13. If I even eat lunch, I do it at my desk while working.

14. I see time as my enemy.

15. I can't tell the difference between work and play; it all feels like one more thing to be done.

16. Everything I do feels like a drain on my energy.

17. I feel like I want to pull the covers over my head and hide.

18. I seem off center, distracted—I do things like walk into mirrored pillars in department stores and excuse myself.

19. I blame my family—because of them, I have to stay in this job and location.

20. I have ruined my relationship with co-workers whom I feel I compete against.

total ☐

Now to interpret the score.

If the number of points you accumulated was in the 20 to 29 area, you're lucky. Your work challenges are normal.

Should your total be in the 30 to 49 range, pressures are becoming a problem. You should try to identify the sources and manage them.

In case your score was over 50, the stressors are dangerously high. You should seek help.

Obviously, the next step is to identify the factors contributing to this unhealthy workplace.

For example, it may be as simple as tobacco. Apropos, there's a great deal of information available to you. If smoking is a problem, you may wish to contact:

Action on Smoking and Health (ASH), 2013 H Street, N. W., Washington, D. C. 20006 (202-659-4310). They provide a guide to a smokefree workplace and other booklets and article reprints free of charge.

The American Cancer Society, 4 West 35th Street, New York, New York 10001, (212-736-3030), can also help you with free smokeout kits for employees.

The Non-Smokers' Rights Association (NSRA) which is headquartered in Canada at Suite 308, 344 Bloor Street, West, Toronto, Ontario, Canada M5S 1W9, (416-928-2900). They offer a free brochure and a purchasable "Smoke in the Workplace Action Kit."

Finally, it may be helpful to refer to the section on smoking elsewhere described (Chapter 15).

But it may not be tobacco...it might well be diet! In this regard, there are many dietary and other nutritional avenues.

For example, a respected asset is the **American Heart Association**, 7320 Greenville Avenue, Dallas, Texas 75231 (214-750-5300). They provide free information on work-related programs and have available for purchase a comprehensive kit called Heart-at-Work.

Why not check your own eating habits by completing the questionnaire in Chapter 14?

When it comes to physical fitness, there's a plethora of printed material available. Specifically, one good place to begin is with the study of absenteeism and work performance as it relates to exercise (p. 180). Secondly, an interesting questionnaire dealing with your physical activity state is described elsewhere (Chapter 17). There are many other useful resources.

For example, the **Association for Fitness in Business (AFB)** promotes employee health and fitness. They publish current data and information through a bimonthly "Action" newsletter, bimonthly research reports and other benefits. They can be contacted at 310 North Alabama, Suite A100, Indianapolis, Indiana 46204 (317-636-6621).

President's Council on Physical Fitness and

Sports, Washington, D. C. 20001 offers free information on fitness in the workplace and a handbook on employee programs.

And let's not forget alcohol. Two excellent contacts are:

Center of Alcohol Studies, Education and Training Division, Busch Campus-Smithers Hall, Rutgers University, Piscataway, New Jersey 08854 (201-932-2190), which offers workplace alcohol abuse prevention information.

The Phoenix House, Drug Education and Prevention Unit, 164 West 74th Street, New York, New York 10023 (212-598-5810) is a national drug abuse organization. It provides free information on work-related drug issues. The unit will assess institutions needs for prevention services and develop programs for supervisors and/or personnel.

But a very good place to begin is to analyze your own drinking habits. You can accomplish this quickly and simply by referring to Chapter 16 entitled **Are You Drinking Too Much Alcohol?**

A panoramic view of the total workplace problem is available by consulting the following organizations:

The American Institute of Stress, 124 Park Avenue, Yonkers, New York 10703, (914-963-1200). They offer free packets.

Human Synergistics, 39819 Plymouth Road,

Plymouth, Michigan 48170 (313-459-1030). This organization is a management consulting firm with stress programs and free information.

For more details concerning interpersonal environments, consult:

National Training Laboratory Institute (NTL), 1240 North Pitt Street, Suite 100, Alexandria, Virginia 22314-1403 (703-548-1500), provides a free brochure on group training for sensitivity. Since its founding in 1947, NTL is known worldwide for its excellence and reliability in human relations training and consultation. Their 1988 brochure lists many unique programs.

Lastly, there are a number of very resourceful organizations devoted to overall wellness programs. They are:

The Center for Corporate Health Promotion, Incorporated, 1850 Centennial Park Drive, Suite 520, Reston, Virginia 22091 (703-391-1900) offers **Taking Care**, an on-the-job program emphasizing lifestyle management and medical self-care.

The Worksite Health Promotion, Office of Disease Prevention and Health Promotion, Switzer Building, 330C Street, S. W., Room 2132, Washington, D. C. 20201 (202-472-5372) will send you a free bibliography of books and organizations.

Finally, you may be interested in a catalog published by **Leisure Press**, a Division of Human Kinetics Publishers, Inc., Box 5076, Champaign, Illinois 61820. They offer books and videos covering various fitness and training categories. Their material is similar to that used by the YMCA.

Lastly, you'll find lots of valuable information in the succeeding bibliography file.

RESOURCES

1. Adamson, G. J.
   Health Promotion and Wellness
   Group Practice Journal 30: #5, 17-22, May/June 1981.

   While there are many trends which are contributing to the rise of health promotion and wellness, this article focuses particularly on two. First, the increasing competition in the health care field. Second, the developing involvement of the corporate sector in the health care experience. This report analyzes these relationships and puts them into modern perspective.

2. Blair, S. N., Piserchia, P. V., Wilbur, C. S., and Crowder, J. H.
   A Public Health Intervention Model for Work-Site Health Promotion: Impact on Exercise and Physical Fitness in a Health Promotion Plan After 24 Months
   Journal of the American Medical Association

This study reports a comprehensive effort to evaluate the sustained effect of a public health intervention model to achieve fitness goals. Employees at four companies were exposed to a health promotion program, while employees at three comparison companies were offered an annual health screen. Daily energy expenditure in vigorous activity increased 104% among employees at companies offering the health promotion program, compared with a 33% rise among employees at comparison companies. Changes in exercise habits were corroborated by estimates of maximal oxygen uptake. Meaningful population changes in exercise and physical fitness can be produced, it is concluded, at the worksite.

3. Bjurstrom, L. A. and Alexious, N. G.
A Program of Heart Disease Intervention for Public Employees
Journal of Occupational Medicine 20: #8, 521-531, August 1978.

A behavior modification program was implemented for characteristically sedentary state employees. Available to workers regardless of age, sex, salary, or health status, the program was supported by federal, state and employee contributions. A formal, 15-week primary intervention consisting of a progressive physical conditioning program was complemented by eight one-hour seminars. An ongoing secondary intervention program reinforced previously incorporated lifestyle modifications and provided an opportunity for further social changes. The five-year experience involving 847 employees resulted in favorable modifications in risk factors, amelioration of health problems and reductions in employee absenteeism.

4. Cohen, S. R.
   Another Look at the In-Plant Occupational Health Program
   Journal of Occupational Medicine 15: #11, 869-873, November 1973.

   The purpose of this report is to define, describe, and defend, where useful, an Occupational Health Program (OHP) that would meet the requirements of acceptable job safety and health care delivery. Included is a discussion of the potential cost-benefit factors of promoting an OHP. Additionally, suggestions are made to deal with deficiencies in work-site health resources as they may be encountered.

5. Cox, N. H. and Shephard, R. J.
   Employee Fitness, Absenteeism and Job Satisfaction.
   Medicine and Science in Sports 11: #1, 105, Spring 1979.

   Twelve hundred and eleven employees of two large Canadian Life Assurance Companies were studied over ten months to determine the effects of an employee fitness program on job satisfaction and absenteeism. One company served as a control, while the other organization acted as the experimental group. Consistent participants (greater than 2 times per week) in the employee fitness program decreased their absenteeism while demonstrating a rise in aerobic power. Absenteeism and aerobic power remained relatively constant in the control company. No changes in job satisfaction were demonstrated at either organization. The data illustrate the positive influence of a well regulated employee fitness program on physical work capacity and absenteeism.

6. Donoghue, S.
The Correlation between Physical Fitness, Absenteeism and Work Performance.
Canadian Journal of Public Health 68: #3, 201-203, May/June 1977.

This is a review of the relationship between these three factors in an attempt to answer the question whether the physically fit employee performs better at the workplace. Utilizing 44 references, the paper demonstrates the existence of a significant positive relationship between physical fitness and absenteeism and physical fitness and work performance. It's concluded that people who are physically fit demonstrate fewer absences due to illness and work significantly more productively.

7. Editors
More Suits Blamed On-the-Job-Stress
Medical World News 27: #8, 118-119, 28 April

1986.

In this article Dr. Paul J. Rosch, President of the American Institute of Stress, is quoted on the health and legal implications of on-the-job stress syndrome. The report emphasizes that this is now a major health problem which is costing industry more than $150 billion a year in terms of absenteeism, reduced productivity, and direct medical expenses. Medical researchers have linked workplace stressors to cardiovascular disease, upper respiratory infections, hypertension, peptic ulcers, migraines, and many other conditions.

8. Ferguson, T.
Contented Workaholics
Medical Self-Care 13: 20-24, Summer 1981.

Workaholics, also called Extra Effort Persons (X-E), as a group are remarkably satisfied with their lives. Unlike the individual who is forced to work long hours at two jobs, the workaholic thrives on work. X-E persons work because the things they love to do most involve working very hard. While workaholics tend to be satisfied with other areas of their lives, they also have a high incidence of burnout, heart disease and family problems. This illuminating article also contains a self-scoring questionnaire to determine whether you are a workaholic.

9. Iglehart, J. K.
Health Policy Report: Health Care and

American Business
New England Journal of Medicine 306: #2, 120-124, January 1982.

American industry, historically a slumbering giant when it comes to influencing the delivery of health-care services that it purchased, has been awakening to the need to become a more sophisticated buyer of such services for one very clear overriding reason (soaring costs are crimping profit margins as never before). Once passive, private businesses began to demonstrate moderate interest in national health issues in the 1970s during debates over federal health insurance, health planning, alternative delivery systems, and medical quality assurance. This report is an excellent historical account of the relationship of health-care and American business.

10. Jennings, C. and Tager, M. J.
Good Health is Good Business
Medical Self-Care 13: 14-18, Summer 1981.

These reporters write a syndicated newspaper column, The Wellness Bag. In this article they discuss the overall trend toward corporate wellness programs interspersed with documentation from specific plans of large corporations such as Xerox, Control Data and others. The authors envision employee wellness programs as a major force for the improvement of the quality of working life. They suggest that business may come to place new emphasis on the health of the workforce, and health workers may learn thrift, accountability and salesmanship.

11. Pelletier, K. R.
Healthy People in Unhealthy Places
1984. New York, Delacorte Press.

Work consumes most of an individual's life for the most critical years and is generally second only to sleep in the actual number of occupied hours. Recently, attitudes toward work have been changing. A propos, the workplace is the most obvious focus when people move from a personal to a collective concern with the determinants of health and longevity. The author takes a hard and unique look at the overall and special problems and the general and specific answers.

12. Stamler, R., Gosch, F. C., Stamler, J., Lindberg, H. A. and Hilker, R. R. J.
A Hypertension Control Program Based on the Workplace
Journal of Occupational Medicine 20: #9, 618-625, September 1978.

In several large Chicago companies and institutions, workplace screening of 7,151 persons yielded 833 suspect hypertensives. Of these, 91% attended a follow-up verification visit, where for 513 persons high diastolic pressure was confirmed. One-half of these people were referred to their physicians for treatment and one-half were randomly assigned to be treated directly by the Hypertension Detection and Follow-Up Program (HDFP) in a step-wise pharmacologic regimen to normalize diastolic pressure. Preliminary experiences in the Chicago Center of the HDFP give encouraging evidence that the workplace is a useful base for successful hypertension control efforts.

11

OTHER PROBLEMS

Clearly, there are many other problems. And obviously they take different forms and shapes. We've talked about problems as symptoms (Chapter 2), looked at problems as disease entities (Chapters 3, 4, and 5), examined problems as biochemical aberrations (Chapters 6 and 7). Problems can also be viewed as states (Chapters 8 and 9). We demonstrated that even the worksite can be a problem (Chapter 10).

It goes without saying that there are more problems than we can deal with. So this chapter will serve as a potpourri, a collection of vignettes.

Let's back up for the moment. We tried to convey the importance of symptomatology with a discussion of America's major so-called **physical** complaint or signal in Chapter 2 (fatigue). It seems now appropriate to dwell on America's number one **mental** presenting symptom.

Depression—that ominous dark cloud that comes in varying shades of grey—is wreaking havoc with the lives of 14 million Americans. In its milder forms, the disease is playing an unusually cruel game of cat and mouse with the emotions of millions more. No wonder it's been dubbed the **common cold** of mental imbalance.

The blues are nothing new, of course. Thousands have suffered depression over the ages, from the Bible's King Saul to First Lady Betty Ford. Even that old taskmaster Sir Winston Churchill fell prey to the gloom that issues forth from somewhere deep inside the mind. The uniqueness of the 80s is that depression is now an epidemic, and from teenage to golden age none is immune.

According to the National Institute of Mental Health (NIMH), the incidence of all kinds of depression is increasing at an alarming rate, with baby boomers representing a large majority of victims. The most recent numbers, culled from surveys across the United States, reveal that one in four women and one in 10 men can expect to suffer a serious bout at some point during their lifetime. Twenty five years ago, the disease erupted mostly in 40-year-olds; today, it's more common in the 20s. Even more disturbing are the estimates of some experts who report depression affects 10 percent of all under-the-age-of-twelve children.

Undoubtably the most tragic side of depression rests on the shoulders of adolescents. The disease not only stunts emotional growth, but in all too many cases robs these young people of precious life by driving them to suicide. The figures show that between 1980 and 1984 adolescent admissions to private psychiatric hospitals increased more than 350 percent, and depression is the most frequently cited reason for the explosion. Shocking!

Suffering from depression, however, doesn't have to be a dead end. Remarkable advances have been made in the last decade which can help pull the depressed person out of the pits and back into the mainstream of life. New drugs, innovative ways of using old pharmaceuticals, recognition of the relationship between diet, exercise and mood, even bold new therapy using light (Reference 6, Chapter 19) to relieve mood disorders, are having a tremendous impact on depression. In fact, experts agree the disease can be significantly relieved in 80 percent of sufferers.

Like any other malady, the real danger when it comes to depression is ignorance. If you don't know what's been making you miserable how can you do anything about it? The affliction is easy to overlook because there are at least a half dozen subtypes, ranging from major unipolar depression (that which lingers for months before lifting) to the seesaw ups and downs of manic depression, otherwise known as bipolar illness. Between theses two extremes there are obvious gradations.

Fortunately, there are scores of superb diagnostic instruments to ferret out the presence and degree of disability. One of the best is the Beck Depression Inventory (BDI) details of which are provided in the bibliographic material at the end of this chapter (p. 202).

For our purpose here a more simple test is provided. It derives from the writings of Frank B.

Minirth, M.D. and Paul D. Meier, M.D. We want to take this time to thank them for allowing us to reproduce their material. More particulars are available in the resource section about their book. Indicate the truth or falsity statements in the appropriate box.

		true	false
1.	I feel like crying more often now than I did a year ago.		
2.	I feel blue and sad.		
3.	I feel hopeless and helpless a good part of the time.		
4.	I have lost a lot of my motivation.		
5.	I have lost interest in things I once enjoyed.		
6.	I have had thoughts recently that life is just not worth living.		
7.	I am losing my appetite.		
8.	My sleep pattern has changed of late. I either sleep too much or too little.		
9.	I am too irritable.		
10.	I am anxious of late.		
11.	I have less energy than usual.		
12.	Morning is the worst part of the day.		

		true	false
13.	I find myself introspecting a lot.	☐	☐
14.	When I look at myself in the mirror, I appear to be sad.	☐	☐
15.	My self-concept is not very good.	☐	☐
16.	I worry much about the past.	☐	☐
17.	I have more physical symptoms (headaches, upset stomach, constipation, rapid heartbeat, etc.) than I did a year ago.	☐	☐
18.	I believe people have noticed that I do not function as well at my job as I did in the past.	☐	☐

The grading is simple. Anyone who answers true to a majority of the above statements is almost certainly depressed and should seek professional assistance.

Regardless of your score, you could benefit from examining and trying some of the therapies listed in the resources section. A good place to start is the book **Feeling Good** by David D. Burns, M.D. (p. 202).

Doctor Burns describes some of the latest scientific methodology for overcoming blue moods and for feeling good about your life. The techniques he recounts are based upon a relatively new form of therapy known as **cognitive treatment**, a fast-acting approach to handling emotional upsets like depression and anxiety. The approach is termed cognitive therapy because it trains you to change the way you look at the world when you're upset and opens the door to feeling better and being more productive. The mood-elevating techniques are relatively simple to master and remarkably effective.

Another approach that is attracting attention is **psychodietetics**. Its roots, psyche and diet, are familiar. The marriage underscores the close relationship between diet and mental health. Once this connection is made clear, proper diet becomes an important tool in the prevention and treatment of mental illness and the principles of psychodietetics apply directly to depression. Check the book **Psychodietetics** (p. 205), particularly the last chapter which deals with the optimal diet and vitamin/mineral supplementation.

Increasingly, many people find that getting their bodies in motion helps beat the blues. But exercise can do even more, as evidenced by a Norwegian study that shows it's also effective for controlling severe depression. Specifically, half of 43 patients hospitalized for major depression in the study had exercise built into their daily routines for nine weeks; the other half served as a control. Those who exercised moderately showed improvement on both mental and physical tests, but the most significant factor was oxygen uptake. The higher the oxygen intake, the greater the antidepressant effect of exercise.

Parenthetic mention should be made that improving nutrition by means of chelating agents can serve as a psychotherapeutic modality. Particulars regarding one such study are outlined in the reference (p. 206).

These as well as other reports on light, demonstrate the burgeoning interest in nonpharmacologic or drug-free modalities of therapy for depression. Common sense, along with preliminary scientific data, suggests that exposure to light may well be one of the critical triggers for that syndrome, which has come to be known as **season affective disorder**, appropriately abbreviated **SAD**. Now psychiatrists at the National Institute of Mental Health have produced reasonably solid evidence to support that hypothesis. They conducted a study of 13 SAD patients during the winter. Six of them were inhouse; the remainder were out-patients. Entry into the study required at least two weeks of continuous depression, as documented by one of the popular testing tools, in this case the Hamilton Rating Scale for Depression. Each patient was treated with one week of exposure to bright light and one seven day period of dim light, separated by a one-week rest period. The researchers found that mood changes seemed to develop within two to four days of starting therapy and regressed over a similar time frame after exposure to bright light was terminated.

Finally, it has long been recognized that certain types of patients regularly slip into depression during winter's gloom (see section on Are you under the Weather in Chapter 19 entitled Other Solutions) and then turn hypermanic during the summer months.

Overall, what's so fascinating is that there's a decrease in the use of drugs for depression and a rise in the awareness of lifestyle as a psychotherapeutic modality. More particulars are available from the references at the end of this chapter and the material in Part C (Solutions).

Now, let's turn to another problem.

Fatigue, as we have observed (p. 19), may well be America's #1 physical **complaint**; depression is surely America's #1 **mental** problem. But we ought not to forget that heart disease is America's #1 **cause of death**.

Did you know:

- In one day—4,100 Americans suffer a heart attack and 1,500 die
- Of every 100 American deaths, 35 are due to heart disease
- There are 500 coronary bypass operations performed each day. This makes it the most common major surgical procedure performed in this country.

If you've obediently (compulsively) been completing the test forms from the beginning (and even the cross-referenced questionnaires) then the next quiz ought not to show any surprises. You'll find that you've already answered just about all of these questions (this may give you an opportunity to check your accuracy!). But the real purpose of this questionnaire at this time is to reframe the queries for a different reason, namely to establish your risk for heart disease.

Take the following six-question quiz developed at Stanford University by John W. Farquhar, M.D. (permission has already been granted to us for citing this form).

Each question may be answered in five different ways and the appropriate score (shown in parenthesis) should be placed in the assigned box. For example, question one deals with cigarette smoking. If you don't smoke, then insert a 0. With up to 9 cigarettes, assign a 1. If you smoke 10 to 24 per day then insert a 2 in the box. A daily consumption of 25 to 34 cigarettes is to be marked with a 3. Finally, 35 or more cigarettes per day should be given a score of 4.

risk habit or factor	your score

I. **smoking cigarettes**
   none per day (0)
   up to 9 per day (1)
   10 to 24 per day (2)
   25 to 34 per day (3)
   35 or more per day (4) ☐

II. **body weight**
   ideal weight (0)
   up to 9 lbs. excess (1)
   10 to 19 lbs. excess (2)
   20 to 29 lbs. excess (3)
   30 lbs. or more excess (4) ☐

III. **salt intake**
   1/5 average—hard to achieve; no added salt, no convenience foods (0)
   1/3 average—no use of salt at table, spare use high-salt foods (1)
   U. S. average—salt in cooking, some salt at table (2)
   above average—frequent salt at table (3)
   far above average—frequent use of salty foods (4) ☐

   or

   blood pressure upper reading (if known)
   less than 110 (0)
   110 to 129 (1)
   130 to 139 (2)
   140 to 149 (3)
   150 or more (4) ☐

IV. **saturated fat and cholesterol intake**
   1/5 average—almost total vegetarian; rare egg yolk, butterfat and

	your score

lean meat (0)

1/3 average—2 meatless days/week, no whole milk products, lean meat only (1)

1/2 average—meat (mostly lean), eggs, cheese 12 times/week, nonfat milk only (2)

U. S. average—meat, cheese, eggs, whole milk 24 times/week (3)

above average—meat, cheese, eggs, whole milk over 24 times/week (4)

☐

or

blood cholesterol level (if known)

less than 150 (0)
150 to 169 (1)
170 to 199 (2)
200 to 219 (3)
220 or more (4)

☐

V. **self-rating of physical activity**

vigorous exercise 4 or more times/week 20 min. each (0)

vigorous exercise 3 times/week 20 min. each (1)

vigorous exercise 1 to 2 times/week (2)

U. S. average—occasional exercise (3)

below average—exercises rarely (4) ☐

or

walking rating

brisk walking 5 times/week 45 min. each (0)

brisk walking 3 times/week 30 min. each (1)

your score

    brisk walking 2 times/week
      30 min. each or
    normal walking 4 1/2 to 6 miles
      daily (2)
    normal walking 2 1/2 to 4 1/2 miles
      daily (3)
    normal walking less than 2 1/2
      miles daily (4)

VI. self-rating of stress and tension
    rarely tense or anxious/ or yoga,
      meditation, or equivalent
      20 min. 2 times/day (0)
    calmer than average/ or feel tense
      about 3 times/week (1)
    U. S. average—feel tense or
      anxious 2 to 3 times/day/ or
      frequent anger or hurried
      feelings (2)
    quite tense—usually rushed/ or
      occasionally take tranquilizer (3)
    extremely tense/ or take tranquilizer
      5 times/week or more (4)

Now total your score and insert the final grade in the box below:

What does all this mean?

Should your score be 21 to 24, the probability of having a heart attack or stroke is about four to five times the United States average. It would be wise to decrease this approximately four points within a month and three more points within six months.

In the case of a grade of 17 to 20, the incidence of

heart attack or stroke is about twice the American average. Try to drop four points within six months and continue reduction.

With a score of 13 to 16 you're within the U. S. average of 14. This is a readily avoidable zone. Careful planning can result in a five- to six-point reduction within a year.

Next, with a grade of 9 to 12 the likelihood of having a heart attack or stroke is about one-half the mean for the country. A reduction of four to six points within the year would be advisable.

In the event of a total of 5 to 8 the incidence of heart attack or stroke is about one-quarter of the United States average. This goal is achievable by many but often takes one or two years to reach.

Finally, with a number 0 to 4, the incidence of heart attack or stroke rates very low averaging less than one-tenth the rate in the United States in the 35 to 65 age group. This goal requires diligent effort, considerable family support, and often takes three to four years. Individuals in this range should be proud and gratified (and will often find themselves acting as models). As a matter of fact, this is the rare kind of person who looks and behaves like he or she is 70 going on 40 in contrast to the more usual individual who is 40 going on 70! This subject will be dealt with at great length in Chapter 20. For the moment, should you wish to examine your risk in greater detail you might refer back to Chapter 6 (How's Your "Good and Bad" Cholesterol?). Also, we would suggest that you examine the bibliographic material at the end of this chapter.

A third and final problem!

As you know, we've been discussing all kinds of problems and have studiously not mentioned **infections**. Who among us hasn't said or heard uttered often "I caught a cold" or "He got the flu" or "She contracted pneumonia?" All of these cliches suggest that one or another microorganism, in someway and somehow not readily understood, has jumped into and overwhelmed the body.

The fact of the matter is that in 1865 (just about a century ago) Louis Pasteur made a discovery from which developed the **germ theory** which has dominated medicine to this day. Once it was known that formerly unheard of **specific** microbes could invade the body and flourish into **specific** diseases, the search to seek out, identify, and combat these villains in our environment was underway. It's by no means ended (to wit, note the forthcoming discussion on yeast).

As one might suspect, the germ theory is convenient and comfortable. Most of us prefer to believe that the illnesses we suffer are the result of external forces—just as we would rather blame bad luck for our failures—like "catching a cold." Phrased another way, the germ theory advocates would have us view man as a helpless quarry eternally trying to elude a multitude of disease-bearing bugs.

It's comforting to note that a relatively small but increasing cadre of medical practitioners, however, has resisted the germ theory as the one simplistic answer to illness. They've carefully noted that while microorganisms are obviously involved in many ailments, their mere presence does not automatically guarantee disease. Three presumably healthy people, for example, can breathe the same germs at the same moment. One may develop pneumonia, another may sniffle his way through a cold, and the third may never be aware that the germs were even there. After all, in the case of most infectious diseases, those people who succumb represent only a fraction of the number of people exposed to them.

Is the germ theory obsolete? Certainly more than one noted scientist now espouses a more sophisticated approach to disease. Doctor G. T. Stewart, Professor of Epidemiology and Pathology at the Schools of Public Health and Medicine at the University of North Carolina, pointed out a long time ago that polio and other viruses can be carried for months with no clinical effect. "The resulting disease," he says, "is in fact determined by the host, rather than the bacillus."

For these and other reasons, we're convinced that just about every disease, physical and mental, is generated by a combination of circumstances which arise both inside and outside the body. It logically follows that illness may be prevented or cured by correcting variables that exist both externally and internally. Simply, we can go after the **germ**, but we can also correct the life conditions which predisposed the individual to illness.

And now to the problem. Do you have a yeast infection?

Answer these 10 questions. (Permission granted by William G. Crook, M.D., The Yeast Connection, 3rd edition, Professional Books, Inc., 681 Skyline Drive, Jackson, Tennessee 38301.)

	yes	no
1. Have you taken repeated "rounds" of antibiotic drugs?		
2. Have you been troubled by premenstrual tension, abdominal pain, menstrual problems, vaginitis, prostatitis, or loss of sexual interest?		

	yes	no

3. Does exposure to tobacco, perfume and other chemical odors provoke moderate to severe symptoms? ☐ ☐

4. Do you crave sugar, breads or alcoholic beverages? ☐ ☐

5. Are you bothered by recurrent digestive symptoms? ☐ ☐

6. Are you bothered by fatigue, depression, poor memory, or "nerves?" ☐ ☐

7. Are you bothered by hives, psoriasis, or other chronic skin rashes? ☐ ☐

8. Have you ever taken birth control pills? ☐ ☐

9. Are you bothered by headaches, muscle and joint pains or incoordination? ☐ ☐

10. Do you feel bad all over, yet the cause hasn't been found? ☐ ☐

Now to the scoring.

If you have 3 or 4 yes answers, yeast **possibly** plays a role in contributing to your problems. With 5 or 6 affirmative responses, yeast **probably** is significant. Should you have 7 or more positive answers, your symptoms are **almost certainly** yeast-connected.

What to do about it? Clearly, there are two avenues. On the one hand utilizing fungicidal agents (such as Nystatin and Nizoral) may be indicated. This obviously requires medical supervision. The other route consists of improving ones' immune responses. This means revamping diet, possibly modifying physical activity, alcohol or tobacco reduction or abstinence and the other lifestyle changes outlined in detail in Section C (Solutions).

For the moment, reference to the two books (pages 205 and 208) in the bibliographic material may be helpful and informative.

RESOURCES

1. Beck, A. T. and Beck, R. W.
   Screening Depressed Patients in Family Practice
   Postgraduate Medicine 52: #12, 81-85, December 1972.

   There's an inherent difficulty in identifying depression even in family practice. Since this finding often masquerades as a somatic disorder and individuals tend to conceal mood deviations, the diagnosis is often overlooked. A sensitive scale has been developed consisting of twenty-one questions. This report describes an abbreviated BDI consisting of only thirteen items showing remarkable correlations with the larger form.

2. Burns, D. D.
   Feeling Good: The New Mood Therapy
   1980. New York, Signet Books.

Some of the latest scientifically tested methods for overcoming blue moods and for establishing good feelings are described in this book. The techniques are based on a relatively new form of treatment known as cognitive therapy, a fast acting approach to handling emotional upsets such as depression and anxiety. Essentially, the treatment is called "cognitive therapy" because the subject is trained how to feel better when upset. The Beck Depression Inventory as well as two other interesting questionnaires are discussed.

3. Cheraskin, E., and Ringsdorf, W. M., Jr.
Electrocardiography and Carbohydrate Metabolism. II. P-Wave Height (Lead I) in Presumably Healthy Young Men
Angiology 21: #1, 18-23, January 1970.

Thirty eight presumably healthy junior dental students participated in this experiment, in which the height of the P-wave in Lead I and blood glucose were determined at 10:00 A.M. on Monday and Friday of the same week. The evidence suggests that the measurement of P_1-wave height is highly reproducible. While the data indicate that blood glucose and the P-wave are inconstant from Monday to Friday, there's a negative and significant correlation between these two parameters. The point of the story is that here's suggestive proof of a subtle electrocardiographic and biochemical connection.

4. Cheraskin, E. and Ringsdorf, W. M., Jr.

Reported Cardiovascular Symptoms and Signs Before and After Dietary Counsel
Alabama Journal of Medical Sciences 9: #2, 174-179, April 1972.

It's clinically well known that heart and blood vessel disease is preceded by a long incubation period. At first, the cardiovascular symptoms and signs are few and diverse. With time, there's an increase in number and more discrete localization. Finally, the findings crystallize and fit the textbook picture which allows a definite classical cardiovascular diagnosis. This report shows that, with advancing age, reported cardiovascular symptoms and signs increase. This study of presumably healthy dentists and their wives also demonstrates that the pattern can be slowed, stopped, and sometimes actually reversed with relatively simple dietary advice.

5. Cheraskin, E. and Ringsdorf, W. M., Jr.
How Much Refined Carbohydrate Should We Eat?
American Laboratory 6: #7, 31-35, July 1974.

It's a fact that refined and unrefined carbohydrate foodstuffs exert different metabolic effects. Notwithstanding, the Food and Nutrition Board of the National Academy of Sciences/National Research Council has made no distinction with their recommendation that the average reference human should be consuming approximately 100 grams of carbohydrate foods. In this report, an attempt has been made to determine a more realistic physiologic requirement through the development of a progressively symptomless and signfree group. Under these conditions, there's presumptive evidence to suggest that, very likely, the optimal daily refined carbohydrate consumption should be approximately zero.

6. Cheraskin, E., Ringsdorf, W. M., Jr., and Brecher, A.
Psychodietetics
1974. New York, Stein and Day (hardback)
1976. New York, Bantam Books (paperback)

Psychodietetics introduces the revolutionary idea that a host of emotional problems, presently labeled mental, including depression, are actually rooted in improper diet and nutrition. The concept that emotional complaints can be prevented, treated, and cured by improved nutrition now hovers somewhere between the stages of ridicule and discussion. This book is primarily an effort to accelerate into general acceptance the principle that food nutrients are an important part of the key to emotional health, so that millions of people, beset by a host of misdiagnosed, nutritionally caused emotional ailments, can benefit.

7. Crook, W. G.
The Yeast Connection, 3rd edition
1986. Jackson, Professional Books

This book is one of two contemporary monographs on the subject of candidiasis. It's especially valuable for lay reading. Of particular interest is its questionnaire (which incidentally is quite elaborate and lengthy and is not included in the text). A ten-question quiz, which will appear in a cookbook presently pending publication, is discussed in this chapter. Parenthetic mention should be made that special emphasis is placed on the role of diet/nutrition in the genesis and treatment of this fungal problem.

8. Farquhar, J. W.
    The American Way of Life Need Not be Hazardous to Your Health
    1978. New York, W. W. Norton & Company

   This book has been cited elsewhere in this monograph because of a quiz regarding physical activity and/or walking (Chapter 17). It's suggested here because of a questionnaire referred to earlier in this chapter dealing with factors in the genesis of heart disease proneness. The test analyzes a number of known contributing factors such as stress, tobacco, weight, and serum cholesterol.

9. McDonagh, E. W., Rudolph, C. J. and Cheraskin, E.
    The Psychotherapeutic Potential of EDTA Chelation
    Journal of Orthomolecular Psychiatry 14: #3, 214-217, Third Quarter 1985.

   This is the only reported experiment designed to ascertain the changes in emotional state following EDTA chelation plus multivitamin/ mineral supplementation. Utilizing one of the respected tests for emotional state, it can be safely stated that the average chelation patient displays significant emotional problems. Following a series of EDTA chelation infusions, the emotional scores are significantly improved. Specifically, there's a reduction in depression of approximately 50%. This underscores the fact that improving nutrition (used in its broadest connotation) serves a possible psychotherapeutic role.

10. Minirth, F. B. and Meier, P. D.
Happiness is a Choice: A Manual on the Symptoms, Causes, and Cures of Depression
1978. Grand Rapids, Baker Book House

This book is up-to-date, clinically thorough, yet nontechnical. It's an easy-to-follow guidebook for families as well as a convenient resource volume for pastors, counselors, and family physicians. These doctors offer basic steps and guidelines for recovering and sustaining a happy, fulfilling and meaningful life. It's included here especially because of a simple questionnaire which is discussed in the text of this chapter.

11. Rippon, J. W.
Medical Mycology, 3rd edition
1988. Philadelphia, W. B. Saunders

It's refreshing to note a medical mycology book that recognizes the correct role of microorganisms in the genesis of health and sickness. The author, a faculty member at Pritzker School of Medicine in Chicago, in a book intended to emphasize the role of fungi in disease, makes it very clear that the microorganism is of secondary importance. Phrased another way, the invasion is only made possible in the face of impaired coping systems.

12. Truss, C. O.
    The Missing Diagnosis
    1983. Birmingham, C. Orian Truss, M.D.

This book represents a popular exposure of the role of Candida albicans to candidiasis. It stems from the author's 20 years of clinical experience with this syndrome. It makes the point that the microorganism is bountiful in nature and in man (particularly the female). It produces diverse symptoms and signs (commonly of a psychologic or psychiatric nature). Finally, the syndrome responds significantly with the reduction or elimination of the fungus and especially in parallel with improvement in the immune response.

12

FINALLY ... ARE YOU A HAPPY PERSON?

I'm sure you'll agree that we've spent lots of time looking at **problems**...in different shapes and sizes... viewed in orthodox systems and unconventional terms. You may have gotten the idea that happiness is simply not being tired, cancer and arthritis-free, and with a good cholesterol and blood sugar, a fat bank account and a great job. All other things being equal, these kinds of people have more reasons to be happy. But it's a mistake to believe that all cancer patients are sad; cancer free persons are glad. It's just not that simple.

And so, we've got to search out who is happy and what it is that makes people happy. At first blush, the definition of happiness is much like the definition of life...it's tough and easier to point at and describe than to define.

As an aside, there's no question the notion of psychologic well-being or happiness has been nagging man since the beginning of time. Indeed, it's been the object of endless thought, discussion and research for many centuries.

That wise old sage Aristotle even addressed the concept when he pronounced "both the general run of men and people of superior refinement say that the highest of all goods achievable by action is happiness ... but with regard to what happiness is they differ, and the many do not give the same account as the wise." For the many, happiness is better translated into the more benign term **well-being**, because Aristotle was interested in more than the pleasurable feelings generally associated with the cliche happiness. In the centuries since Aristotle the terms of the debate may have changed somewhat, but there continues to be agreement that happiness or well-being appears to be the goal of man's action and there's still discord between the **many** and the **wise** concerning what makes people happy.

And so, what is happiness really?

Science has been struggling with that very question for years. Some within the psychosocial community think happiness is the ability to adjust to a world about and within us. And so it figures, these same scientists believe that maladjustment constitutes unhappiness. In some corners this maladaptation has even been equated with mental illness. Surely there are circumstances in which being happy would be inappropriate and perhaps even a sign of psychologic imbalance. The person who derives joy from others' suffering for example. Would you call that person healthy mentally? So if you're not particularly happy at the moment, it doesn't mean you're going off the deep end. The fact is many of us only think we know what will make us happy. Over and over again we've all heard this chant from friends: "I'd be happy as a lark if I had a million dollars." Would they really?

To find out what makes people happy, two reputable psychologists put their heads together and conducted a massive survey in an attempt to get to the root of that age old question. You may find the results surprising.

In 1975, Philip Shaver as an Associate Professor of Psychology at New York University joined forces with Jonathan Freedman, a Professor of Psychology at Columbia University. The two arranged a graduate seminar and invited students to examine that which they felt was important. They chose **happiness**. The group designed a questionnaire and it was this form which appeared in the October 1975 issue of Psychology Today. About a year later, the magazine published results of the findings from 52,000 readers, ranging in age from 15 to 95. Before we get to some of the specifics and the conclusions, it must be underlined that these respondents were on the average, younger, more affluent, better educated and more liberal than the average middle American. Hence, generalizations to all Americans must be guarded. Also keep in mind the age-old warning that people who willingly complete a survey are clearly more interested in the topic than those who don't.

What did we learn? Lots! In general, those who answered the questionnaire fell into two catagories. One group looked upon happiness as the usual state and believed sorrow is a fleeting interlude. For the others, happiness is the exception that life is a bunch of battles and bruises, and it only comes occasionally.

To hone in on more specifics, the readers were queried about happiness in sixteen different life experience areas. For single folks, being happy with one's friends, work, lovelife and level of recognition represented the most cardinal contributions to overall happiness. With married couples, the issues are somewhat different and even varied between the sexes. A wife's fundamental happiness, for instance, comes from her satisfaction with love, marriage, her husband's happiness and her sex life, pretty much in that order. With the married man, personal growth and development rates tops followed by love, marriage, work, and the wife's happiness in that sequence.

Surprisingly, issues that seem to contribute little to happiness are also noteworthy. For example, satisfaction with one's physical attractiveness is really not very important, though single people are more concerned about it than marrieds. And, believe it or not, religion doesn't contribute much to happiness for either single or married respondents, according to the Psychology Today survey.

Just a few more vignettes: the women with the best of all possible worlds seem to be those who are married and employed outside the home; sexual satisfaction comes from quality, not quantity; sexual problems are unrelated to overall happiness in men; the happiest are those in love with partners who love them equally; few childhood experiences contributed with any reliability to adult happiness; people who live in the city and in the country are equally happy, or unhappy; and at least among Psychology Today readers, education, work, and income are not the critical keys to contentment.

There's, however, general agreement among investigators in this field that an individual's position on the scale of psychologic well-being may be mapped out in terms of two poles. One may be pictured as positive affect (emotion) and the other at the opposite extreme negative affect (emotion).

This model specifies that a person will be high in psychologic well-being depending on the degree to which he or she shows an excess of pluses/minuses, and will be low in well-being to the extent to which negative affect (NA) predominates over positive affect (PA). It's clear from this model that these two dimensions are independent of one another, which makes it impossible to predict an individual's score on the negative affect parameter from any knowledge of his or her score on the positive range and vice versa. However, both characteristics are related in the expected direction to overall self-ratings of happiness or subjective well-being. In fact, the best predictor of the overall self-rating is the discrepancy between the two scores: the more positives one has than negatives means the overall rating of psychologic well-being is greater.

As you might expect, there are lots of **happiness** tests. Some are listed in the resource section. They all have virtues and limitations. One of the more sophisticated and most recent is the Memorial University of Newfoundland Scale of Happiness, commonly referred to by its acronym MUNSH. We acknowledge with gratitude permission granted to us by Doctors Albert Kozma and Michael J. Stones to cite here this questionnaire.

Before we go on to anymore discussion about the general topic of happiness, try the MUNSH test. The questions describe how things have been going in recent days. Complete this twenty-four question form using the following grading system. (There are two exceptions. Question #14 asks about where you live. If you like where you are presently living, answer with a 2, if you prefer some other location, assign 0. A propos, question #16, regarding life satisfaction, if you are satisfied, insert 2; not pleased, place 0.)

statement is not true = 0
don't know = 1
statement is true = 2

1. On top of the world? (PA)

2. In high spirits? (PA)

3. Particularly content with your life? (PA)

4. Lucky? (PA)

5. Generally satisfied with the way your life has turned out? (PA)

6. Bored? (NA)

7. Very lonely or remote from other people (NA)

8. Depressed or very unhappy? (NA)

9. Flustered because you didn't know what was expected of you? (NA)

10. Bitter about the way your life has turned out? (NA)

11. I am just as happy as when I was younger. (PE) ☐

12. The things I do are as interesting to me as they ever were. (PE) ☐

13. As I look back on my life, I am fairly well satisfied. (PE) ☐

14. If you could live where you wanted, where would you live? (PE) ☐

15. I am as happy now as I was when I was younger. (PE) ☐

16. How satisfied are you with your life today? (PE) ☐

17. My health is the same or better than most people's my age. (PE) ☐

18. This is the dreariest time of my life. (NE) ☐

19. Most of the things I do are boring or monotonous. (NE) ☐

20. Things are getting worse as I get older. (NE) ☐

21. Feel lonely a lot? (NE) ☐

22. Little things bother me more this year. (NE) ☐

23. I sometimes feel that life isn't

worth living. (NE) ☐

24. Life is hard for me most of the time. (NE) ☐

Reexamine questions 1, 2, 3, 4, and 5 (you'll note they are marked by PA) and you'll find a common denominator of positive affect. They are the pluses which were mentioned earlier.

Add these scores. The lower limit could be 0; the upper 10. Now place your total PA in the box.

☐ **Positive Affect**

Now turn your attention to questions 6, 7, 8, 9 and 10 (marked as NA) which have negativity as a common denominator. These are the minuses we discussed earlier. Once again, the limits are from 0 to 10. Add the scores and insert in the square below:

☐ **Negative Affect**

Now turn your attention to the last 14 questions which relate to more general life experiences. Questions 11 through 17 (marked PE) are of a positive nature. These answers are to be summed and the range will extend from 0 to 14. Place your total in the box.

☐ **Positive Experience**

Questions 18 through 24 (designated NE) collectively are the minuses. Put this score in the appropriate place:

☐ **Negative Experience**

Now, you're ready to derive an overall happiness score, a total MUNSH, by taking the PA minus the NA plus the PE minus the NE. The highest possible score is +24 and this signifies the top happiness grade; the lowest attainable number is -24 and it represents the maximal unhappiness level.

$$\boxed{} - \boxed{} + \boxed{} - \boxed{} = \boxed{}$$
PA **NA** **PE** **NE** total happiness score

Are you **happy** with your score?

If not, the mere inventory that you've just completed may indicate simple changes you can make to improve it, like altering a place to live or work or seeking out less boring tasks. On the other hand, there may be a real need for aptitude testing and/or counselling. Perhaps, there's a food-mood connection, that could be adjusted by referring to the book **Psychodietetics** listed in the resource section. Also, you may wish to check the dietary questionnaire in the next section (Chapter 14).

An addendum...

We should have listened. Edward Arlington Robinson warned us over fifty years ago in his marvelous poem about the rich and good-looking Richard Cory who had everything money could buy... yet went home and put a bullet through his head!

Angus Campbell, Director of the University of Michigan's Institute for Social Research, looked into the Richard Cory syndrome to ferret out the relative importance of income and education as it contributes to one's well-being. First, he discovered what had already been known, that the sense of **health and happiness** increases as people earn more money and get better education. (So, you might wish to go back and check your **financial health** on p. 151.)

But there were lots of surprises. All other things being equal, "The happiest people in the country are those who did not finish high school but who are earning more than $12,000 a year . . . their accomplishments outdistanced their expectations . . . college graduates, on the other hand, are not especially happy no matter how much they earn. Possibly the expectations of college grads have outstripped their accomplishments."

There's obviously much more to this fascinating area. Perhaps glancing through the resources may help clarify special and individual problems.

RESOURCES

1. A Questionnaire
   What Makes You Happy?
   Psychology Today 66-72, October 1975.

   This survey was designed to pinpoint the meaning of happiness, when one feels it, what one thinks will bring it about, why one does or doesn't have it, how it relates to personality and past. Researchers at Columbia University have been pondering these questions and suggested that Psychology Today readers might well provide the answers. Hence, the survey was designed by professors Jonathan Freedman and Phillip Shaver along with their staffs. It's the most contemporary questionnaire intended to answer the question, "What makes you happy?"

2. Abramson, M., Angers, W., Cherepon, J., Kohut, M. and Lalouch, H.
   Pilot Analysis of a Happiness Questionnaire

Psychological Reports 48: 570, 1981.

A research team conducted an extensive statistical analysis of the Angers Happiness Questionnaire, a 10-item self-rating form in which were reported demographic measures and subjects' self-perceptions of their individual happiness, as well as the quality of their interpersonal relationships. Over a 1-year period, 600 questionnaires were administered. Of these, a sample of 125 was drawn to reflect a wide range of demographic factors such as age, marital status, occupation, and educational level. Multiple regression analyses showed that interpersonal relationships, frequency of happiness, age, and marital status affected the question "Are you happy?". Thus, people who reported that they were happy tended to be older, married, and satisfied with their interpersonal relationships.

3. Bradburn, N. N. and Caplovitz, D.
Reports on Happiness
1965. Chicago, Aldine Publishing Company

Happiness and its correlates are the ambitiously conceived subjects of the researches reported in this volume. This is not an attempt to uncover the causes of happiness. Rather, it's constructed to see how self-assessments of happiness are distributed throughout the social groupings of the American population and how the American people vary over time in its level of happiness. Reports on happiness consolidates two of the initial studies in this continuing program. This research began in 1961 when the National Institute of Mental Health entered into a contract with the National Opinion Research Center (NORC) for the design and development of prototype instruments that would measure fluctuations in behavior related to mental health.

4. Cheraskin, E., Ringsdorf, W. M., Jr., and Brecher, A.
Psychodietetics
1974. New York, Stein and Day (hardback)
1976. New York, Bantam Books (paperback)

This lay text attempts to analyze the food-and-mood connection and considers a spectrum of behavioral expressions ranging from depression and happiness to schizophrenia in terms of overall eating habits along with single and combinations of vitamins and minerals.

5. Kozma, A. and Stones, M. J.
The Measurement of Happiness: Development of the Memorial University of Newfoundland Scale of Happiness (MUNSH)
Journal of Gerontology 35: #6, 906-912, November 1980.

Two Canadian psychologists started with three commonly used happiness questionnaires, the Affect Balance Scale, the Life Satisfaction Index-Z, and the Philadelphia Geriatric Center Scale, and developed a new 24 item questionnaire (the one utilized in this chapter). The results suggest that the new scale, the MUNSH, is a better predictor of avowed happiness than existing testing techniques.

6. Kozma, A. and Stones, M. J.
   Re-Validation of the Memorial University of Newfoundland Scale of Happiness
   Canadian Journal of Aging 2: #1, 27-29, March 1983.

   The present investigation represents a re-validation of the Memorial University of Newfoundland Scale of Happiness (MUNSH) and its Negative (NAS) and Positive Affect (PAS) subscales in an institutionalized sample of elderly urban residents. Self-ratings of happiness versus judges' ratings were used as criteria measures. The findings indicate that the MUNSH is as valid for residents of large urban centers as for the smaller institutions in which it was initially developed.

7. Kozma, A. and Stones, M. J.
   Predictors of Happiness
   Journal of Gerontology 38: #5, 626-628, September 1983.

   This report deals with the temporal stability of happiness as analyzed by the Memorial University of Newfoundland Scale of Happiness (MUNSH) and the stability of the predictor/happiness relationships in three subgroups of persons over 64 years of age. The respondents were interviewed twice, 18 months apart, on the

MUNSH and on nine established correlates. The results show that, although predictor effectiveness may differ across subgroups, happiness, as measured by this particular questionnaire, remains reasonably stable.

8. Shaver, P. and Freedman, J.
   Your Pursuit of Happiness
   Psychology Today 10: #3, 26-32, 75, August 1976.

   This fascinating survey disclosed what more than 52,000 readers of Psychology Today (ranging in age from 15 to 95), feel and know about happiness. They indicated that money can't buy happiness, unhappy children frequently grow up to be happy adults, sexual satisfaction is more qualitative than quantitative, atheists are as happy, or unhappy, as church-goers.

9. Wood, V., Wylie, M. L. and Sheafor, B.
   An Analysis of a Short Self-Report Measure of Life Satisfaction: Correlation with Rater Judgments
   Journal of Gerontology 24: #4, 465-469, October 1969.

   This paper reports the relationship between two measures of life satisfaction or morale based on ratings made by trained judges versus a direct self-report instrument. These techniques were developed in the Kansas City Study of Adult Life. The evidence suggests a statistically significant correlation.

C

THE SOLUTIONS

Now that we've dragged out your problems, where do we go? There are two options. First, conventional wisdom dictates that discrete diseases require discrete treatment plans. Thus, for example, we've recounted that traditional thinking recognizes most cancer is best handled with surgery, radiation, and/or chemotherapy. On the other hand, the treatment of choice, as we've discovered, for the majority of the arthritides is aspirin, gold therapy, and the steroids. Implied, if not stated, is that the cancer treatment couldn't possibly help the arthritic; the arthritis regime isn't indicated for cancer.

But, after a sobering interlude, common sense suggests otherwise.

For the moment, there's also an obvious continuing nature (genetic) versus nurture (environmental) debate. It recognizes these two elements in the causation of problems.

Secondly, it should be evident from the last section, that there are common therapeutic denominators for all diseases. We may have discovered that what's **good** for arthritis may well be **good** for cancer. Conversely, what's **bad** for arthritis is also probably **bad** for cancer. This common characteristic springs from lifestyle. And lifestyle embraces pretty much the air we breathe, the water we drink, the food we eat, and the thoughts we think.

The forthcoming chapters will view first our lifestyle in general terms (Chapter 13) and then will hone in on more particulars.

13

HOW FANTASTIC ARE YOU?

Believe it or not, there's lots more to lifestyle than most of us think. We've made it sound like our way of life simply embraces the air we breathe, the water we drink, and the food we eat. The fact of the matter is that our lifestyle includes scores of behavioral patterns which, at first blush, one would not consider to be part of our personal social system.

You should have guessed it. We even brought it to your attention. Remember the section on bank account (Chapter 9) and workplace (Chapter 10)? There's no question...these areas mold our way of life.

But there's still more...much more.
- Have you considered the role of friends and their contribution to your health and happiness?
- Did you ever wonder where the telephone fits in your lifestyle?
- Are you willing to admit that, as a coffee consumer, you're really a drug taker?
- What is the significance of positive thinking?
- What happens when you can no longer drive a car?

As we've just learned, there's lots **of** lifestyle. Additionally, there's also lots **to** lifestyle.

One recent United States Government report, entitled **Healthy People: The Surgeon-General's Report of Health Promotion and Disease Prevention**, acknowledged the importance of recognizing manageable events. They flatly state: "It is the controllability of many risks—and often the significance of controlling even a few—that lies at the heart of disease prevention and health promotion."

In the final analysis, these risk factors consist of a series of pluses and a bunch of minuses. The positive ones are desirable and encourage **health and happiness**; the negatives invite disease. So, what we have is a collection of antagonistic forces. **Health and happiness** is represented by a predominance of pluses; illness by a majority of minuses.

We'd be remiss in not offering you a relatively easy way to spot these pluses and minuses. Assessing lifestyle factors over which you have at least some degree of control is the quickest way. The following questionnaire does just that in **broad strokes**.

The FANTASTIC Lifestyle Assessment Inventory, was developed by Douglas M. C. Wilson, M.D., of McMaster University in Canada, and has been widely used by physicians. This is a very good time for us to thank Professor Wilson for allowing us the privilege of reprinting this exciting form. Don't be fooled by its simplicity, FANTASTIC has proven to be a surprisingly comprehensive instrument in assessing lifestyle and identifying areas which could be affecting your **health and happiness.** Try it!

FANTASTIC is an acronym with each letter representing a different area of lifestyle. **Based on the past month**, rate yourself in each of the areas. Circle the correct answer. Grade yourself using the number of points shown at the top of each column.

	2 points	1 point	0 points

The **F** stands for **family** and **friends**.
1. I have someone to talk to about things that are important to me. — almost always / some of the time / hardly ever

2. I give and I receive affection. — almost always / some of the time / hardly ever

The **A** represents **activity**.
1. I am physically active (gardening, climbing stairs, walking, housework). — almost always / some of the time / hardly ever

2. I actively exercise for at least 20 minutes (running, cycling, fast walk). — 4 times or more per week / 1-3 times per week / less than once per week

The **N** relates to **nutrition**.
1. I eat a balanced diet,

		almost always	some of the time	hardly ever
	(foods from the basic four food groups).			
2.	I often eat excess sugar or salt or animal fats or junk foods.	none of these	some of these	all of these
3.	I am within ____ lbs. of my ideal weight.	10 lbs (4 kg)	20 lbs (8 kg)	not within 20 lbs.

The **T** designates **tobacco** and **toxics**.

1.	I smoke tobacco.	not in past 5 years	not in past year	have smoked in past year
2.	I usually smoke ____ cigarettes per day.	none	5-10	more than 10
3.	I use drugs such as marijuana, cocaine.	never	occasionally	fairly often
4.	I overuse prescribed or "over the counter" drugs.	never	occasionally	fairly often
5.	I drink caffeine-containing coffee, tea, or cola.	less than 3 per day	3-6 per day	more than 6 per day

The **A** signals **alcohol**.

1.	My average alcohol intake per week is (1 drink = 10 oz. bottle/ /beer, 4.5 oz. glass/wine, 1.25 oz. shot/spirits).	0-7	8-13	more than 14

2. I drink more than four drinks on an occasion. never   occasionally   fairly often

3. I drive after drinking. never   only rarely   fairly often

The S signifies **sleep, seatbelts** and **stress**.

1. I sleep well and feel rested. almost always   some of the time   hardly ever

2. I use seatbelts. always   some of the time   hardly ever

3. I am able to cope with the stresses in my life. almost always   some of the time   hardly ever

4. I relax and enjoy leisure time. almost always   some of the time   hardly ever

The T portrays **type of personality**.

1. I seem to be in a hurry. hardly ever   some of the time   fairly often

2. I feel angry or hostile. hardly ever   some of the time   fairly often

The I describes **insight**.

1. I am a positive or optimistic thinker. almost always   some of the time   hardly ever

2. I feel tense or uptight. hardly ever   some of the time   fairly often

3. I feel sad or depressed. hardly ever   some of the time   fairly often

The **C** connotes **career**.

1. I am satisfied with my job or role.   almost always   some of the time   hardly ever

total score ☐

Multiply by 2

total fantastic percentage ☐

What's this number mean?

If your grade is 85 to 100%, congratulations, you've got a good handle! In other words, you have a pretty healthy lifestyle.

With a score of 70 to 84%, good work—you're on the right track.

The range of 60 to 69% means fair.

In the incidence of 40 to 59%, you had better take more control—which means change your ways. This might be a good time to reexamine your pluses and minuses in this quiz. For example, if this superficial accounting suggests poor dieting, you might begin by examining the next chapter. This, in a sense, will pin point your specific nutritional problems.

Finally, 0 to 39% signals danger—but honesty is your real strength!

We've all heard of the ages of man...traditionally viewed in seven stages. You may not have heard that the **new** look is three...the young, the old, and you're lookin' great!

There's lots of good reasons for reexamining the FANTASTIC concept in the young versus the aging. There are significantly different questions to be asked and, as you might expect, there are significantly different answers.

If you're in the ages of 14 to 18, you might wish

to complete the following form. Rate yourself in each area which best describes your behavior or situation **in the past month**. Circle the correct answer. Grade yourself using the number of points shown at the top of each column. Parenthetic mention should be made at this time that while the overall design of the teenager form is like the earlier general questionnaire, there are some appropriate differences.

	2 points	1 point	0 points

The **F** is for **family** and **friends**.

1. I have a friend to talk to about things that are important to me. — almost always / sometimes / hardly ever

2. I get along well with my family (parents, brothers, sisters). — almost always / sometimes / hardly ever

3. I am satisfied with my relationships with friends of the opposite sex. — almost always / sometimes / hardly ever

(You'll note that these F questions for the teenager are different than those for the overall population.)

The **A** describes **activity**.

1. I actively exercise for 20 min. (running, cycling, swimming) outside of physical education classes. — 5 or more times/week / 3 times/week / less than once/week

The **N** expresses **nutrition**.

1. I eat balanced meals (foods from the basic four food groups). — almost always / sometimes / hardly ever

2. I often eat excess salt or animal fats or junk foods. — none of these / some of these / all of these

3. My weight is: — okay for me / slightly over or under / very over or under

The **T** relates to **tobacco** and **toxics**.

1. I use tobacco. — never / occasionally / almost daily

2. I use street drugs. — never / occasionally / almost daily

The **A** applies to **alcohol**.

1. I drink alcohol (e.g. 1 drink = 10 oz. bottle/beer, 4.5 oz. glass/wine, 1.25 oz. shot/spirits). — never / occasionally / almost daily

2. I drink more than 4 drinks on an occasion. — never / rarely / fairly often

3. I drive after drinking and/or ride with a driver who has been drinking. — never / rarely / fairly often

The **S** speaks to **sexuality**, **safety** and **stress** (You will note the S is different from the original.)

1. If I were sexually active, I would use a reliable method of preventing infection. always usually rarely

2. I would use a reliable method of birth control. always usually rarely

3. I use seatbelts. all of the time sometimes never

4. I obey the rules of the road when walking, riding or driving (wear helmet when riding motorcycle, face the traffic when walking). almost always sometimes almost never

5. I follow safety rules when involved in sports activities (water, team or racquet). almost always sometimes almost never

6. I sleep well and feel rested. almost always sometimes almost never

The **T** portrays **today** and **tomorrow**.

1. I am satisfied with my school work. almost always sometimes hardly ever

2. I think about my future career choices. often sometimes never

The **I** expresses **identity** and **independence**.

1. I like myself as a person. almost always some of the time almost never

2. I have a reasonable amount of freedom.   almost always   some of the time   almost never

The **C** conotes **crisis** and **coping**.

1. I feel life is not worth living.   never   sometimes   almost always

2. I think of killing myself.   almost never   sometimes   almost always

3. When I have a problem, I am able to solve it.   almost always   sometimes   almost never

total score ☐

Multiply by 2

total fantastic percentage ☐

What does this grade mean?

Should your score be 85 to 100%, congratulations—you're in control!

With a grade of 70 to 84%, good work—you're on the right track.

A total of 60 to 69% is considered fair.

The 40 to 59% range, is recognized as somewhat low—you must make changes! This is a good time to reexamine the pluses and minuses in this quiz.

If you score in the 0 to 39% category, you're in the danger zone (but honesty is your real strength!)

Now if you're one of those who's lookin' great, Doctor Wilson has provided you with a different FANTASTIC form. You'll find that this questionnaire varies both from the overall original and the teenage form. Should you qualify, fill it out.

Rate yourself in each area which best describes

your behavior or situation **in the past month**. Circle the answer that applies to you. Remember, there are no right or wrong responses. Just be honest!

	Column 1	Column 2	Column 3

F, as in the other two questionnaires, represents **family** and **friends**.

1. I have someone to talk to about things important to me. — almost always / sometimes / hardly ever

2. I give and I receive affection. — almost always / sometimes / hardly ever

3. I see my family at least: — weekly / monthly / hardly ever

A stands for **alone** and **activity**.

1. I feel lonely. — hardly ever / sometimes / always

2. I am physically active (gardening, housework, exercises, walking). — almost always / sometimes / hardly ever

3. I participate in social activities (church, cards, small groups). — weekly / monthly / hardly ever

N represents **nutrition**.

1. I eat balanced meals (e.g. from the basic four food groups). — daily / some days / hardly ever

2. My weight is: okay for me / slightly over or under / greatly over or under

3. I often eat excess sugar, salt, animal fats, junk food. — none of these / some of these / all of these

T denotes tobacco and toxics.
1. I smoke tobacco. — not in past 5 years / not in past year / have smoked in past year

2. I overuse prescription or non-prescription drugs. — never / occasionally / fairly

A describes alcohol.
1. My average alcohol intake per week is: (e.g. 1 drink = 10 oz. bottle/beer, 4.5 oz. glass/wine, 1.25 oz. shot/spirits). — 0-7 / 8-13 / more than 14

2. I drive after drinking or with a drinking driver. — never / only rarely / fairly often

S signifies sleep and stress.
1. I sleep well and feel rested. — almost always / sometimes / hardly ever

2. I feel able to cope with the stresses in my life. — almost always / sometimes / hardly ever

T relates to **telephone, transaction** and **travel**.

1. I use the telephone. — daily / 3 times/week / less than once/week

2. I can manage my own money. — almost always / sometimes / hardly ever

3. I have a lawyer and a will. — both / 1 of the two / neither

4. I use taxi, public transportation or drive. — almost always / sometimes / hardly ever

5. I use seatbelts. — almost always / sometimes / hardly ever

I portrays **insight**.

1. I feel useful and needed. — almost always / sometimes / hardly ever

2. I feel tense or uptight. — hardly ever / sometimes / fairly often

3. I feel sad or depressed. — hardly ever / sometimes / fairly often

C conotes **care** and **control**.

1. I forget to take my medicines. — hardly ever / sometimes / fairly often

2. I make my own decisions. — almost always / sometimes / hardly ever

What's this checklist mean?

For the circles you have in Column 1, congratulations—you have lots of pluses!

You're on the right track for the times you circled Column 2—but you can improve even more by adding pluses or subtracting minuses.

Should you have made any circles in Column 3, this is a somewhat low grade—you should think about making some changes in your daily life habits but do it wisely. In other words, add the pluses and subtract the minuses slowly.

Something else needs discussion. It should be pretty obvious from earlier portions of this book and especially this chapter that we think the environment is the all-important solution to our many problems. Not true. The multifactorial matrix, the nature (genetics) versus nurture (environment) debate is still very much alive. Just this year (1988) two of the most distinguished scientific periodicals (Nature and The New England Journal of Medicine) published articles and editorials on this topic. They proclaim (and we agree) that both inheritance and our lifestyle determine our **health and happiness**. What they have studiously avoided is assigning relative importance to nature versus nurture. By act, if not in print, the buzzword is **familial**. The assumption is that what's familial is necessarily inherited. Surely, in many instances, this is true (Chinese parents produce Chinese children). But it's possible that familial means just that...it runs in the family and may in part or exclusively be environmental or genetic.

We've been looking at this issue for a long time...prompted by the sometimes cliche suggesting that **if you live with her long enough you'll look like her**. In other words, there's a familial model which cannot be genetic (since the average male doesn't marry kin).

As a matter of fact, we're not the only ones who have been looking at this problem in a somewhat creative system. Professor R. B. Zojonc at the University of Michigan and his colleagues submitted separate photographs of men and women to his psychology class students. They were asked to match up married couples. It was extremely difficult to pair recently married husbands and wives; the predictability was extraordinary in the married couples of long standing. As an aside, the investigators conclude that, with time, the physical appearance increased significantly supporting the old cliche that couples begin to look alike after a number of years of living together (even pets begin to resemble their masters!).

Apropos, we've published approximately 20 papers dealing with spouse likeness ranging from studies of actual physical appearance, clinical state, biochemical patterns, and even enzymes. While there are some obvious minor differences, in general, regardless of the parameters examined, three points were evident. First, husbands and wives show similar patterns. Secondly, this is not apparent at the time of marriage. Thirdly, the correlations become clear with time, usually after 15 years of cohabitation.

If indeed this is true, and it seems to be so from our work and that of others (Stanley Garn), then it heightens and sharpens the importance of nurture over nature. For more particulars, check references #2 and #3 of ours and #4 of Garn's in the bibliographic material.

And there's another practical correlary if all this is true, then you might want to have your spouse take these quizzes.

Now returning to our findings, the good news is that in this chapter you now have some idea of your lifestyle habits. The not-so-good news is that the appraisal may be relatively shallow. In other words, you may sense that smoking or alcohol may be a serious lifestyle problem. If so, check these matters. The chapters which follow provide some magnification of your social habits.

Now before you proceed to the other areas dealing with individual lifestyle parameters, we'd suggest that you examine the succeeding bibliographic material.

RESOURCES

1. Bertera, R. L.
   How Fit are You?
   Modern Maturity 46-47, August-September 1986.

   About two thirds of all major illness and premature death in the U. S. are linked to lifestyle. The social habits of a hypothetical 62-year-old American male are presented. They include weight, smoking, alcohol consumption, blood pressure, drugs, stress, exercise, cholesterol, nutrition, highway safety (seat belts), and medical checkups. Using the data collected from these questions, it's possible to predict how long this theoretical creature will live. A self-rated longevity questionnaire is included.

2. Cheraskin, E.
   Risk Factors or Risk Indicators?
   Proceedings of the Sixth International Conference on Human Functioning, Wichita, Kansas, September 1982. p. 91-105.

   Health and happiness hinges on a battery

of risk analyses. These may be further categorized as primary risk factors and secondary risk indicators. The primary elements are those variables which directly contribute to health and sickness (e.g. tobacco, alcohol, physical activity). The secondary group influence wellness indirectly (e.g. blood pressure, serum cholesterol). Finally, both sets of variables may be categorized as pluses (dedicated to health promotion) versus minuses (designed to encourage disease.)

3. Cheraskin, E., Ringsdorf, W. M., Jr., and Medford, F. H.
Familial Enzymic Patterns: III. Serum Glutamic Oxalacetic Transaminase (SGOT) in the Dentist and His Wife (Final Report)
Nutrition Reports International 12: #1, 35-40, July 1975.

It's frequently assumed that familial patterns are genetically dominant. One hundred eighty-two dental practitioners and their spouses were studied in terms of serum glutamic oxalacetic transaminase (SGOT). The data reveal a statistically significant correlation between the husbands and the wives. Thus, this study corroborates an earlier smaller experiment with 48 couples, that environmental influences undoubtedly play a major role in enzyme patterns since married couples are rarely genetically related.

4. Garn, S. M., Block, W. D., and Solomon, M.A.
Lipids and Living Together

American Journal of Clinical Nutrition 33: #7, 1714-1715, July 1980.

Doctor Garn and his associates summarized in this report their observations in other areas as well as their new findings. Sequential cholesterol determinations were made on some 12,000 participants in the Tecumseh Community Health Study of the University of Michigan. The findings with cholesterol in this study underscore their many other observations supporting the similarities of spouse likeness.

5. Lander, E. S.
Splitting Schizophrenia
Nature 336: #6195, 105-106, 10 November 1988.

It has long been known that schizophrenia shows a tendency to cluster in families. In contrast to a one percent lifetime risk of schizophrenia in the general population, the risk has been estimated at about ten percent for a first-degree relative of a schizophrenic and 50 percent for an identical twin. Of course, familial clustering is not synonymous with genetic inheritance. Exposure of family members to a common environment has been suggested to play an important role. A leading hypothesis in the 1960s identified the causative agent as overbearing mothers. In the 1970s, genetic explanations gained favour. While the author does not resolve the problem, he tends to lean toward genetics with his psychiatric demonstrations.

6. Pauling, L.
How to Live Longer and Feel Better
1986. New York, W. H. Freeman and Company.

    Dr. Pauling states that it is possible to live longer and extend your years of well-being by following the advice he offers in this book. This two-time Nobel Prize winner whose research into the healing effects of vitamin C has received worldwide attention, continues to suggest that individuals consume critical amounts (usually larger than recommended) of vitamin supplements. "Moreover, it is now possible to take these important nutrients in optimum amounts, far larger than can be obtained in foods, and in this way to achieve a sort of superhealth, far beyond what was possible in earlier times." This volume, particularly the vitamin regimen it contains, is a valuable resource for those wishing to live longer, healthier lives.

7. Shealy, C. N.
Total Life Stress and Symptomatology
Journal of Holistic Medicine 6: #2, 112-129, Fall/Winter 1984.

    Dr. Shealy, a past president of the American Holistic Medical Association, presents the Total Life Stress Test. This form is designed to ascertain the effect of emotional, chemical and physical stressors. It's achieved by comparing a Total Life Stress (TLS) score with the overall number of symptoms an individual has.

8. Sherk, C., Thomas, H., Wilson, D. M. C. and Evans, C. E.
Health Consequences of Selected Lifestyle Factors: A Review of the Evidence, Part II.
Canadian Family Physician 31: 129-139, January 1985.

This is the last in a series of seven articles designed to validate the utility of the FANTASTIC questionnaire. One of the prime virtues of this quiz is that it can provide information quickly. The lifestyle practices that it assesses include physical, emotional and social factors that influence mortality, morbidity and quality of life. The evidence of the relationship between these lifestyle factors and health is more compelling for some elements than others (e. g. tobacco consumption and seatbelt use).

9. Williams, R. R.
Nature, Nurture, and Family Predisposition
New England Journal of Medicine 318: #12, 769-771, 24 March 1988.

This Letter-to-the-Editor is worthy of careful scrutiny for three reasons. Firstly, it underscores the fact that, even in 1988, there's still a debate raging regarding genetics versus environmental influences in health and sickness. Secondly, this report is a companion to a similar document which appeared in this same year in another prestigious journal (Nature). Finally, it's evident that there's still a reluctance to assign the relative influences of nature versus nurture in the area of health and happiness.

10. Wilson, D. M. C. and Ciliska, D.
Lifestyle Assessment: Development and Use of the FANTASTIC Checklist
Canadian Family Physician 30: 1527-1532, July 1984.

There's no question but that one important aspect of health promotion is the assessment of lifestyle factors over which patients have some control. This article, the first in a seven-part series on lifestyle assessment, describes the development and rationale of a simple patient questionnaire called FANTASTIC (the one used in this chapter.) This was originally intended as a mnemonic memory aid for patients and physicians in the Department of Family Medicine at McMaster University.

11. Zajonc, R. B., Adelmann, P. K., Murphy, S. T. and Niedenthal, P.M.
Convergence in the Physical Appearance of Spouses
Motivation and Emotion 11: #4, 335-346, 1987.

This study attempted to determine whether people who live with each other for a long period of time grow physically similar in their facial features. Photographs of couples when they were first married and 25 years later were judged for physical similarity and for the likelihood that they were married. The results showed that there's indeed an increase in apparent similarity after 25 years of cohabitation. Among the explanations of this phenomenon that were examined, one based on a theory of emotional efference emerged as promising. This theory proposes that emotional processes produce vascular changes that are, in part, regulated by facial musculature. The facial muscles are said to act as ligatures on veins and arteries, and they thereby are able to divert blood from, or direct blood to, the brain. An implication of the vascular theory of emotional efference is that habitual use of facial musculature may permanently affect the physical features of the face.

14

**HOW
WELL
DO
YOU
EAT?**

Did you know:
- The average American eats one teaspoon of artificial colors, flavors, and preservatives daily which adds up to almost four pounds a year?
- In one day, we buy more than one million boxes of Cracker Jacks?
- Every man, woman and child in this country averages eating 2 teaspoons of sugar per day?

Is it any wonder that in the U. S. A. each day:
- 4100 Americans suffer a heart attack.

- 126 lose their eyesight.
- 2200 discover they have cancer and 1000 die.

And we've already, in earlier chapters, provided lots of other relevant mortality and morbidity statistics.

What's important is that there's increasing evidence that the so-called balanced America diet plays a significant role in many disease patterns. For example, we've already pointed out the reasonably scientific facts for the connection between diet and cancer (Chapter 3). There's a plethora of proof indicating that the consumption of large amounts of animal fat can contribute to heart disease (Chapter 6). As a matter of fact, there are lots of studies showing nutritional connections from the womb to the tomb. Should you wish more corroboration check **Diet and Disease** in the suggested reading (p. 264).

Let's face the facts, just because you get three squares a day doesn't mean you're eating well. After all, it's a prepackaged, sugar-coated, salt-laden, grease-drenched world of culinary delights we live in, and a full stomach cannot automatically be equated with a good diet.

So how do you determine whether your eating habits are good or bad? At best it's difficult. The most sophisticated technique is to be locked away in a metabolic ward where all that you eat and drink and everything you excrete is carefully measured over a several-day period. But these shenanigans are clearly cumbersome and expensive. The alternatives or the trade-offs are relatively simple questionnaires which can be dumped into a computer to reveal more than an inkling of your dietary habits. Some of them can actually be self-administered and even self-scored.

The one coming up fits that category. (Reprinted

from **Nutrition Action Healthletter** which is available from the Center for Science in the Public Interest, 1501 16th Street, N.W., Washington, D.C. 20036, for $19.95 for 10 issues, copyright 1986.)

You'll note that there are 30 questions which focus on cardinal features of your diet. Put your scores in the appropriate boxes. The final grade will give you some idea of how good or bad you're eating. Provide one answer to each question.

1. How many times per week do you eat unprocessed red meat? (Include steak, roast beef, lamb or pork chops, burgers, etc.)
    (a) 1 or less   +3
    (b) 2-3   +2
    (c) 4-5   -1
    (d) 6 or more   -3

2. Do you trim the visible fat off red meat?
    (a) yes   +3
    (b) no   -3
    (c) don't eat meat   +3

3. How many times per week do you eat processed meats? (Include hot dogs, bacon, sausage, bologna, luncheon meats, etc.)
    (a) none   +3
    (b) 1-2   +2
    (c) 3-4   -1
    (d) 5 or more   -3

4. What type of bread do you usually eat?
    (a) whole wheat   +3
    (b) rye   +2
    (c) pumpernickel   +2
    (d) white or wheat   -2

5. How many times per month do you eat deep-fried foods? (include fish, chicken, vegetables, potatoes, corn or potato chips, etc.)
   (a) none   +3
   (b) 1-2   0
   (c) 3-4   -1
   (d) 5 or more   -3   ☐

6. How many servings of vegetables do you usually eat per day? (One serving = 1/2 cup. Include potatoes.)
   (a) none   -3
   (b) 1   0
   (c) 2   +1
   (d) 3   +2
   (e) 4 or more   +3   ☐

7. How many servings of cruciferous vegetables do you usually eat per week? (One serving = 1/2 cup. Count only kale, broccoli, cauliflower, cabbage, brussels sprouts, greens, bok choy, kohlrabi, turnip, rutabaga.)
   (a) none   -3
   (b) 1-3   +1
   (c) 4-6   +2
   (d) 7 or more   +3   ☐

8. How many servings of vitamin A-rich fruits or vegetables do you usually eat per week? (One serving = 1/2 cup. Count only carrots, pumpkin, sweet potatoes, cantaloupe, spinach, winter squash, greens, apricots, broccoli.)
   (a) none   -3
   (b) 1-3   +1
   (c) 4-6   +2
   (d) 7 or more   +3   ☐

9. How many times per week do you eat at a fast-food restaurant? (Include burgers, fried fish or chicken, croissant or biscuit sandwiches, topped potatoes, and other main dishes. Omit meals containing plain baked potato and salad only.)
   (a) none   +3
   (b) 1   0
   (c) 2   -1
   (d) 3   -2
   (e) 4 or more   -3

10. How many grains rich in complex carbohydrates do you eat per day? (One serving = 1 slice of bread, 1 large pancake, or 1/2 cup cooked cereal, rice, pasta, bulgar, wheat berries, kasha, or millet. Omit heavily sweetened cold cereal.)
    (a) none   -3
    (b) 1-2   0
    (c) 3-4   +1
    (d) 5-6   +2
    (e) 7 or more   +3

11. How many servings of beer, wine, or liquor do you drink? (Count as one serving: 12 oz. regular or light beer or 4 oz. wine or 1 oz. liquor.)
    (a) 1 or less a week   +3
    (b) 2-3 a week   +1
    (c) 4-6 a week   -1
    (d) 1-2 a day   -2
    (e) more than 2 a day   -3

12. How many times per week do you eat fish or shellfish? (Omit deep-fried items, tuna packed in oil, mayonnaise-laden tuna salad—a little mayo is okay.)
    (a) none   -2

    (b)   1-2   +1
    (c)   3-4   +2
    (d)   5 or more   +3

13. How many times per week do you eat cheese? (Exclude low-fat cottage cheese. Include pizza, cheeseburgers, veal parmigiana, cream cheese, etc.)
    - (a)   1 or less   +2
    - (b)   2-3   +1
    - (c)   4-5   -2
    - (d)   6 or more   -3

14. How many servings of fresh fruit or juice do you consume per day? (One serving = 1 piece of fruit or 6 to 8 ounces of juice.)
    - (a)   none   -3
    - (b)   1   0
    - (c)   2   +1
    - (d)   3   +2
    - (e)   4 or more   +3

15. Do you remove the skin before eating poultry?
    - (a)   yes   +3
    - (b)   no   -3
    - (c)   don't eat poultry +3

16. What do you usually put on your bread or toast? (Average two or more if necessary.)
    - (a)   butter   -3
    - (b)   cream cheese   -3
    - (c)   margarine   -2
    - (d)   diet margarine -1
    - (e)   jam   0
    - (f)   fruit butter   +3
    - (g)   just your lips   +3

17. Which of these beverages do you drink on a typical day? (Average two or more if necessary.)
    (a) fruit juice   +3
    (b) water or club soda   +3
    (c) diet soda   -1
    (d) coffee or tea   -1
    (e) soda or fruit drink   -3

18. How many servings of caffeine-containing beverages do you drink per day? (One serving = 1 cup coffee, tea or 12 oz. cola.)
    (a) none   +3
    (b) 1   +1
    (c) 2   -1
    (d) 3   -2
    (e) 4 or more   -3

19. Which flavorings do you most frequently add to foods? (Average two or more if necessary.)
    (a) garlic or lemon juice +3
    (b) herbs or spices   +3
    (c) soy sauce   -2
    (d) salt   -3
    (e) nothing   +3

20. What do you eat most frequently as a snack? (Average two or more if necessary.)
    (a) fruit or vegetables   +3
    (b) sweetened yogurt   +2
    (c) nuts   -1
    (d) chips   -2
    (e) cookies   -2
    (f) granola bar   -2
    (g) candy bar   -3
    (h) pastry   -3
    (i) nothing   0

21. What is your most typical breakfast?
    - (a) croissant or doughnut   -3
    - (b) eggs and toast   -3
    - (c) coffee or nothing   -2
    - (d) refined cereal or toast   -1
    - (e) whole grain cereal or toast   +3

22. What do you usually eat for dessert? (Average two or more if necessary.)
    - (a) pie or cake   -3
    - (b) ice cream   -3
    - (c) yogurt, ice milk, or fruit ice   +1
    - (d) fruit   +3
    - (e) none   +3

23. How many times per week do you eat beans, split peas, or lentils?
    - (a) none   -1
    - (b) 1   +1
    - (c) 2   +2
    - (d) 3 or more   +3

24. What kind of milk do you drink?
    - (a) whole   -2
    - (b) 2% lowfat   0
    - (c) 1% lowfat   +2
    - (d) 1/2% or skim   +3
    - (e) none   0

25. Other than fresh vegetables, fruit, and beans, what did you choose the last time you ate at a salad bar? (Add two or more if necessary.)
    - (a) nothing, lemon, vinegar   +3
    - (b) reduced-calorie dressing   +1

    (c) regular dressing   -1
    (d) croutons, bacon bits   -1
    (e) cole slaw, pasta salad, potato salad   -1

26. What sandwich fillings do you eat most frequently? (Average two or more if necessary.)
    (a) luncheon meat   -3
    (b) cheese   -1
    (c) peanut butter   +1
    (d) tuna or salmon   +3
    (e) chicken or turkey   +3

27. What do you usually spread on sandwiches?
    (a) mayonnaise   -2
    (b) light mayonnaise   -1
    (c) mustard   0
    (d) ketchup   0
    (e) nothing   +3

28. How many egg yolks do you eat per week? (Include quiche.)
    (a) 2 or less   +3
    (b) 3-4   +2
    (c) 5-6   -1
    (d) 7 or more   -3

29. How many times per week do you consume canned or dried soups? (Omit low-sodium soups.)
    (a) none   +3
    (b) 1-2   0
    (c) 3-4   -2
    (d) 5 or more   -3

30. How many servings of a rich source of calcium do

you eat per day? (One serving = 2/3 cup milk, yogurt; 1 oz. cheese; 1 1/2 oz. sardines; 3 oz. salmon; 5 oz. tofu; 1 cup greens, broccoli; 200 mg. of calcium supplement.)

(a) none   -3
(b) 1   +1
(c) 2   +2
(d) 3 or more   +3

total score

your grand total:

+89 to +51 **great!**   You get a gold star and a pound of collard greens.

+50 to +21 **good**   Pin your Quiz to a wall or bulletin board (with your name in large print, of course.)

+20 to -10 **fair**

-11 to -84 **poor**   Empty your refrigerator and cupboards, and start over.

Seriously, if you fell into the fair or poor category, you need help, and here's where to find it.

The Human Nutrition Information Service, U.S. Department of Agriculture, can provide dietary guidelines and a list of materials on how to use them. Write to Room 325A, Federal Building, Hyattsville, Maryland 20782.

Additional assistance with questions concerning diet and health can be obtained by communicating with Consumer Inquiries, Food and Drug Administration, 5600 Fishers Lane, Rockville, Maryland 20857.

If you can't wait, then contact the dietitian, home

economist or nutritionist at one of the following groups in your area: Public Health Department, County Extension Service, State or Local Medical Society, American Red Cross Chapter, Dietetic, the Diabetes and/or the Heart Association or the nearest Health Center or Clinic.

In addition to those listed above, the resources section of this chapter offers some excellent suggested reading material that can help you, and in many cases may actually show you, how to improve existing medical problems by dietary means. For example, should the orthodox resources now seem inadequate, you might check the more orthomolecular possibilities as outlined by Doctor Ruth Yale Long (reference #10).

You may want to hone in on some specifics in your eating habits. For example, there are dietary surveys intended to isolate foods that contribute to mental health and sickness. Should you wish such information we refer you to the Alpha Test (p. 268).

Remember, we cautioned that there is no perfect questionnaire. The form used earlier developed by CSPI is as good as any other general dietary record survey. However, it does have its limitations. For example, its approach to dietary cholesterol differs somewhat from our earlier discussion (Chapter 6).

An interesting set of quizzes has been developed by Sandra Gordon Stoltz and published in an exciting book entitled **The Food Fix**. Unfortunately, some of her material is too cumbersome to utilize here. However, it is cited at the end of this chapter (p. 269).

It should be recalled that, in the beginning of this section, mention was made of sugar consumption. For example, you may be interested to learn that at the time of George Washington, the average American's annual consumption of sugar was two pounds. At the turn of this century, people in the United States ingested approximately 50 pounds of sugar per year per person. Today, it's about 120 pounds per annum. This translates into about 20 teaspoonsful of sugar per day per person.

Because of this inordinate amount and the fact that the CSPI questionnaire didn't focus on this particular problem, you might wish to take the following test. It will provide you with some measure of the consequences of sugar intake. (This material reproduced from **The Food Fix** by Sandra Gordon Stoltz, copyright 1983 and reprinted by permission of the publisher, Prentice-Hall, Inc., Englewood Cliffs, N.J.)

Rate each statement on a scale of 4 to 0 as follows: 4 = usually, 3 = frequently, 2 = sometimes, 1 = rarely, 0 = never.

1. Do you eat quantities of sweets and processed carbohydrates; cereals, bread, crackers, baked goods, chips, pretzels, candy, and soft drinks?

2. Do you lust after sweets? Are your hungers often specifically for sweets or processed carbohydrates?

3. Do you experience a rush of energy, a "high" or a similar stimulating response when you eat sweets?

4. Do you notice a mood change after eating sugar or foods containing sugar?

5. Does a sugar binge leave you enervated, depressed, or irritable several hours later or the next day?

6. Do you get sleepy within two to four hours after eating manufactured carbohydrates?

7. Do your cravings for and actual consumption of food increase after you eat foods that contain sugar?

8. Do you often eat sweets or processed carbohydrates instead of a nutritious meal?

9. Do you experience withdrawal symptoms—headache, shakiness, achiness, hot and cold spells, lethargy, insomnia—when you abstain from your sugary and starchy confections?

10. After going without all sugar and refined starches for at least a week, do you feel like a different person?

11. Do you eat sweets in secret?

12. Would you feel ashamed if others knew of your total sweets consumption?

13. Do you also shock yourself when you tally up several days' intake?

14. Do you arrange your life around getting a supply of sweets? For example: shopping at the grocery store that has the freshest, most appealing doughnuts; talking the office crew into lunching at the pie shop; shopping for candy bargains the day after Christmas, Easter, or Valentine's Day.

15. Do you cover your addiction by peddling your drug to others? Examples: keeping the candy dish on your desk filled for the boss and your co-workers; buying or baking sweets for co-workers, your family, or neighbors on every possible occasion and inventing a few new occasions; invariably including desserts, even at a wine and cheese party, a brunch, or a cocktail party.

sugar total

If your score was 22 or above, a carbohydrate intolerance or an allergic reaction to specific foods may be contributing to your food cravings and destructive eating.

Before we close this chapter, there are items which have been mentioned but must be underlined. There are other areas which should be checked off briefly.

The point has been made and should be underscored that dietary surveys only assess food intake and, at best, do it quite crudely. The hope, by utilizing several quizzes (as in this chapter) is that the end result will approach greater completeness.

But let's get it straight. Dietary quizzes don't reckon with other nutritional considerations. By dietary analysis, we learn nothing about absorption, assimilation, utilization and excretion. All of these processes play a cardinal role in ultimate cellular nutrition. Fortunately, there are now available at the research level and even in commercial circles nutritional tests. These largely consist of measures of certain vitamins and minerals in the blood.

Next, we must admit that just about nothing has been mentioned about fluid intake. (We'll be looking at this issue in Chapter 19). However, it's well to say here and now that it should be of great concern. In some circles it's recognized that dehydration may well be one of, if not the most, significant factor in geriatric **health and happiness**. Without embarking on a big discussion, the general concensus is that most of us would be well-served by drinking six to eight glasses of good water each day.

It's interesting that the principal thrust thus far has been on **what** to eat. Nothing has been said regarding **when** to eat. There are studies which address this topic. You might check the work of Doctor Paul Fabry published in Lancet and abstracted at the end of this chapter. He shows, as have others, unequivocal evidence of the benefits of eating smaller amounts more frequently. For example, if one were to consume one sixth of the food six times in a given day that one ordinarily eats one third of thrice daily, the clinical and physiologic benefits would be unbelievable. For example, there would be when indicated, weight loss, reduction in serum cholesterol, and an improvement in the glucose tolerance pattern.

Finally, you may recall, we introduced the nature-nurture debate in the last chapter. It was pointed out the scope of spouse likeness underlining that it is even demonstrable at the enzyme level. Our spouse studies have also extended to the eating habits of husbands and wives in terms of calories, carbohydrates, proteins, and fats. There's no question but that spouses, with time together even begin to eat the same. It's reported in the resource section with regard to vitamin A consumption (p. 262).

On a more practical note if indeed our observations are correct, then you might want to have your spouse take these questionnaires.

Now to the suggested readings.

RESOURCES

1. Brody, J.
Jane Brody's Nutrition Book
1981. New York, Norton.

   The author, who is the New York Times' personal health columnist explores nutrition from A to Z, including breast feeding, the best foods for those engaged in sports and weight loss. Ms. Brody also gives advice of strategies for good health and provides a wealth of government agencies, industry groups and even universities where the reader can get orthodox assistance.

2. Cheraskin, E. and Ringsdorf, W. M., Jr.
Familial Dietary Patterns: Daily Vitamin A Consumption in the Dentist and His Wife
International Journal for Vitamin Research 40: #2, 125-130, 1970.

Eighty-two dental practitioners, 82 wives, and 82 women (wives of other dentists) age-paired with the wives, were studied in terms of daily vitamin A consumption. A comparison of the samples suggests that there's only a statistically significant correlation in the married couples. The results are very similar to the findings with regard to daily total calories, total and refined carbohydrates, fat, and total and animal protein. With advancing age, the vitamin A consumption correlation in the married couples is exceeded only by the intake of total and refined carbohydrate foodstuffs.

3. Cheraskin, E. and Ringsdorf, W. M., Jr.
How much Refined Carbohydrate Should We Eat?
American Laboratory 6: #7, 31-35, July 1974.

It is a fact that refined and unrefined carbohydrate foodstuffs exert different metabolic effects. Notwithstanding, the Food and Nutrition Board of the National Academy of Sciences/National Research Council makes no distinction with their recommendation that the average adult should be consuming approximately 100 grams of carbohydrate foods. An attempt has been made to determine a more realistic physiologic requirement through the development of a progressively symptomless and sign-free group. Under these conditions, there's presumptive evidence to suggest that, very likely, the optimal daily refined carbohydrate consumption should be approximately zero.

4. Cheraskin, E., Ringsdorf, W.M., Jr., Clark, J.W.
   Diet and Disease
   1975 (Fifth Printing). Emmaus, Rodale Press (hardback)
   1988. New Canaan, Keats Publishing, Inc. (paperback)

   According to the Council on Foods and Nutrition of the American Medical Association, dated 13 July 1970, "America is now aware that malnutrition is here...In all likelihood, malnutrition is much more prevalent than hunger per se, but it is not as politically dramatic...Malnutrition producing physiologic impairment is probably common..." This citation formed the basis of a discussion of the relationship of diet and nutrition and especially vitamins and minerals to the common killing and crippling diseases ranging from the common cold to cancer.

5. Cheraskin, E., Ringsdorf, W. M., Jr, Medford, F. H., and Hicks, B. S.
   The "Ideal" Unrefined Carbohydrate Intake
   Journal of the American Society of Preventive Dentistry 7: #1, 6-7, January-February 1977.

   Under the conditions of this experiment, approximately 147 grams of unrefined carbohydrates may be designated as the ideal daily allowance. This is noteworthy in view of the fact that the Food and Nutrition Board simply recommends at least 50 to 100 grams of carbohydrates with no consideration as to whether the carbohydrate foodstuffs are refined or unrefined. The technique utilized here provides a mechanism and a goal not previously considered.

6. Connor, S. and Conner, W. E.
The New American Diet
1986. New York, Simon & Schuster

This book is based on the five-year study of 233 American families that was sponsored by the National Institutes of Health and supervised by the authors. The cardinal purpose for including this text here is the unusual in-depth questionnaire which is available for those who wish to self-administer and self-score their own eating habits in a fairly sophisticated system.

7. Fabry, P., Fodor, J., Hejl, Z., Braun, T., Zuolankova, K.
The Frequency of Meals: Its Relation to Hypercholesterolemia and Decreased Glucose Tolerance
Lancet 2: #7360, 614-615, 19 September 1964.

This report is intended to show by means of a carefully-designed experiment the importance of food frequency. All subjects received precisely the same quality and quantity of food per day. In one group, one third of the food was consumed three times a day. In others one fourth four times during the 24-hour period. Other groups were given part of the food as in between meal or bedtime snacks. However dispensed, the evidence is clear that every clinical and biochemical parameter studied improved as the amount of food consumed per session was decreased and more sessions were added.

8. Hoffer, A.
Orthomolecular Medicine for Physicians
1989. New Canaan, Keats Publishing Company

This book is probably the most recent attempt to define and describe orthomolecular medicine. It's authored by a distinguished practitioner and researcher. While the text has been designed for physician use, it's highly readable and can serve well in the hands of the sophisticated layman. Among its numerous unique features is that it's well-referenced.

9. Leveille, G., Zabik, M. E. and Morgan, K. J.
Food Facts: Nutrients in Food
1984. Cambridge, The Nutrition Guild

The nutritional composition of almost 3,000 foods is presented along with a list of about 60 nutrient factors. Unlike many other texts, the authors actually list the nutritional composition of foods by brand name—Big Mac, Nabisco potato chips, Hostess Twinkies, etc. An extensive overview of the Required Daily Allowances (RDAs) is also presented.

10. Long, R. Y.
The Official Nutrition Education Association Home Study Course in The New Nutri-

tion
1989. New Canaan, Keats Publishing Company

There are many well-established and traditional texts designed to provide lay and professional information regarding diet and nutrition. Some of the agencies cited in this chapter can provide adequate bibliographic avenues for obtaining such information. On the other hand, there are also many texts intended to provide alternative opinions regarding foods and food habits. The author has provided here an up-to-date accounting of the general subject and interesting subsets. For example, chapters are included dealing with diet and mental problems, allergies, children's problems and especially diet in relationship to learning and behavior.

11. Marks, J.
A Guide to the Vitamins: Their Role in Health and Disease
1975. Lancaster, MTP Medical and Technical Publishing Co., Ltd.

Dr. Marks reviews the present state of knowledge regarding the value and importance of vitamins. It's designed as an introduction to the subject for doctors, medical students and nutritionists. The biochemical and physiologic states within the body that result from vitamin deficiencies are discussed, as well as ensuing disease states. Numerous tables and photographs are included.

12. Pfeiffer, C. C., Mailloux, R. and Forsythe, L.
    The Schizophrenias: Ours to Conquer
    1988. Wichita, Bio-Communications Press.

   There are many questionnaires designed to relate the general diet to general health and sickness. There are very few forms intended to show the associations between specific eating habits and specific health problems. The Easy Alpha Test, developed by Carl Pfeiffer and his associates at the Brain-Bio Center, is an excellent example of a questionnaire intended to correlate specific nutrients and specific emotional problems. At the moment, this is probably the only questionnaire that looks into the association between, for example, depression in young people and nutritional factors.

13. Staff of Prevention Magazine
    The Complete Book of Vitamins
    1977. Emmaus, Rodale Press.

   This is undoubtedly one of the most comprehensive easy-to-read books ever written on vitamins. Topics include the best food sources for each vitamin; guidelines for spotting vitamin deficiencies; how to get the most for your money when buying vitamin supplements; the role of vitamins in preventing heart disease, cancer and emotional problems; a nutritional approach to hayfever; vitamins for autistic children and much, much more. There are charts that list each vitamin, their major activity in the body, primary sources, clinical deficiency signs and preventive or therapeutic applications.

14. Stoltz, S. G.
    The Food Fix
    1983. Englewood Cliffs, Prentice-Hall, Inc.

    This exciting book offers an innovative approach to solving foodaholic behavior. Increasingly, experts are recognizing that food is or at least may be likened to a drug. This book will help you become responsible for your own health and eating patterns. It provides a litany of techniques to deal with the emotions involved in destructive eating. Included are several informative questionnaires. One, unfortunately long and cumbersome will not be used here. However, the reader may find it revealing. Another very short form is incorporated in this text because it pin points the problem of refined carbohydrate consumption.

15. Trowell, H., Burkitt, D. and Heaton, K.
    Dietary Fibre, Fibre-depleted Foods and Disease
    1985. London, Academic Press.

    A comprehensive view of the fibre connection in human disease is discussed. The authors, who are well-established experts actively engaged in dietary fiber research, explore the alleged hazards of eating fiber depleted foods. Other chapters present the implications of fiber for mineral and energy metabolism, milling and fiber, along with proposals and prospects for a better Western diet.

15

WHY DO YOU (REALLY) SMOKE?

- one out of every 4 Americans smokes cigarettes
- the average tobacco consumer smokes a cigarette every 30 minutes
- we spend $8 billion a year treating smoke-related diseases
- it translates into (according to health economists at the University of California) a nickel every hour round the clock for all of us (smokers and nonsmokers)

In short, notwithstanding the recent and successful educational campaigns netting a significant decline in tobacco consumption, smoking continues to be a big problem.

How damaging is it?
- a cigarette smoker is 10 times more likely to get lung cancer than a nonsmoker
- cigarette smoking contributes to hardening of the arteries in 1 out of 3 cases
- it's estimated that lifespan is reduced 5 1/2 minutes for each cigarette smoked
- projected productivity and earnings loss amounts to 37 billion dollars annually

Clearly, there are widespread ravages stemming from tobacco intake. Phrased another way, this is so because nicotine and other smoking products are protoplasmic poisons, which is a fancy way of saying that tobacco is deadly to cells—all cells. It's our prediction that, if and when tobacco is studied with the same enthusiasm, time and money now being spent on AIDS or artificial heart transplants, one point will become evident. Since all cells are damaged by nicotine and some of its byproducts, then all diseases are influenced by smoking in some way.

And by the way, there's the obvious assumption that there are two kinds of people: smokers and nonsmokers. Actually, there are three categories. The first includes those who clearly smoke (the smoking smokers). There's a second group (probably smaller than we think) who truly do not smoke (the nonsmoking nonsmokers). Finally, there's a very large group who, at first blush, seem to be nonsmokers. However, these are individuals who live with or work with or in some other way associate with smokers. These are actually smoking nonsmokers or nonsmoking smokers (depending upon the way you wish to label them).

- In a smoky room a nonsmoker could inhale enough nicotine and carbon monoxide in an hour to have the same effect as having smoked a whole cigarette.
- The nonsmoking wives of smokers die four years earlier than the nonsmoking wives of nonsmokers.
- The children of smokers score lower in psychologic testing. They're also more hyperactive.
- Kids whose mothers smoked 10 cigarettes a day or more during pregnancy proved to be shorter, and were three to five months behind the offspring of nonsmokers in reading, mathematics, and general ability.

In short, the evidence cited here along with much more not quoted tells us that tobacco consumption is truly dangerous and of pandemic proportions!

Let's put it another way. We've all heard of the two inevitables...death and taxes. From what has just been outlined, there's a third, namely, tobacco. One way or another (actively or passively) just about everybody is a smoker!

Fortunately, there's good news.
- About 10 years after kicking the habit, the death risk to an exsmoker is nearly the same as that of someone who never smoked.
- Nonsmoking men tend to show a stronger drive for achievement.
- Interestingly, high income males smoke less than men in the low income group.

But the burning question facing this nation is: Why do people smoke? Do you smoke because you're nervous? Or are you nervous because you smoke?

Smoking and emotional difficulties are likely to keep each other going. A number of British researchers have discovered that heavy smoking creates a desire for caffeine and sugar. Here's something to think about:

- smokers drink far more coffee, heavily sugared, than nonsmokers
- twice as many smokers have been found among alcohol drinkers than among nondrinkers.

In combination, caffeine, nicotine, alcohol, and refined sugar may well put a tremendous strain on the body's ability to control blood glucose level, and this may indeed increase the potential for emotional disturbances. For more particulars, check the chapter on low blood sugar (p. 109).

So, once again, why do you smoke? What do you get out of smoking? Are you hooked on nicotine?

Here are eighteen statements made by smokers describing what they get, or think they get, out of cigarettes. We gratefully acknowledge permission granted to us by the American Cancer Society to reprint it.

You'll note that each statement can be answered in five ways. Five indicates always; 4 signifies frequently; 3 means occasionally; 2 represents seldom and 1 is to be used for never. For example, if your answer to the first question "I smoke cigarettes to keep myself from slowing down" is always then place a 5 in the box; if the reply is never insert a 0.

Now to the first question.

1. I smoke cigarettes to keep myself from slowing down.

2. I smoke to stimulate me, to perk me up.

3. I smoke cigarettes to give me a lift.

Now add the scores from these three questions and insert in the box.

☐ = **stimulation**

A total score of 11 or above is high; scores of 7 or below is low. (This grading will be used throughout this questionnaire.)

If you score high on this factor, it suggests that you're one of those smokers who is stimulated by the cigarette—you feel that it helps wake you up, organize your energies, and keep you going. For you, physical activity like walking, swimming, playing tennis or running could be a useful substitute. Check Chapter 17 on exercise.

Let's ask more questions:

4. Handling a cigarette is part of the enjoyment of smoking. ☐

5. Part of the enjoyment comes from the steps I take to light up. ☐

6. Part of the enjoyment is watching the smoke. ☐

As in the earlier instance (and this will be the foremat for the rest of this test), add the totals for these three questions:

☐ = **handling**

If this number is high (namely 11+), then fondling things appears to be satisfying. There are many ways to keep your hands busy without lighting up or playing with a cigarette. Did you know, for example, women tend to smoke more while talking on the telephone than at any other time?

There is still a third way of looking at the problem:

7. Smoking cigarettes is pleasant and relaxing.

8. I find cigarettes pleasurable.

9. I want a cigarette most when comfortable, relaxed.

☐ = **relaxation**

It's not always easy to ascertain whether you use cigarettes to feel well; that is, derive real, honest pleasure out of smoking (and this is what we're talking about when we say relaxation) or to keep from feeling bad which will be the next item to be discussed (tension). About two-thirds of those who take this test score high or fairly high on accentuation of pleasure, and about half of these also score as high or higher on reduction or negative feelings. Those who indeed derive real pleasure out of smoking often find that an honest and forthright consideration of the harmful effects of their habit is generally enough to help them quit.

But, in many cases, the problem is not one of relaxation but of tension.

10. I light up when I feel angry about something.

11. When I feel uncomfortable or upset, I light up.

12. When I feel blue, or want to take my mind off cares and worries, I smoke cigarettes.

☐ = **tension**

Many smokers use the cigarette as a crutch in

moments of stress or discomfort. But the heavy smoker, the individual who tries to handle severe personal problems by smoking many times a day, is apt to discover that cigarettes don't effectively help cope with tension. In this case, physical activity serves as an excellent substitute. Once again, refer to Chapter 17.

Now to the area currently receiving the greatest attention.

13. When out of cigarettes, I find it almost unbearable until I can get them. ☐

14. I am very aware of the fact when I am not smoking. ☐

15. I get a real gnawing hunger for a cigarette when I haven't smoked for a while. ☐

☐ = **addiction**

Quitting smoking is difficult for those who scored high on this factor. For them, the craving for the next cigarette begins to build up the moment one is snuffed out, so tapering off is not likely to work. This is the one situation that warrants **cold turkey**. It may be helpful to smoke more than usual for a day or two, so that the taste for cigarettes is spoiled, and then stay completely away from cigarettes until the craving has vanished. Parenthetic mention should be made regarding the United States Surgeon General Koop's just-released report...which recognizes beyond question that tobacco is one of the most addictive habits and probably as serious as heroin and cocaine.

And finally, there is a routinization of smoking.
16. I smoke automatically without

even being aware of it.

17. I light up without realizing I still have one burning.

18. I've found a cigarette is in my mouth and didn't remember putting it there.

☐ = **habit**

Smokers who fall in this category no longer get much satisfaction from cigarettes. They just light up without even realizing what they are doing. For them, kicking the habit may be simply a matter of becoming aware of each cigarette smoked. On the other hand, changing habits may require more complex motivation. For example, there's evidence to indicate (p. 284) that the average 40-year old woman who smokes shows facial wrinkles of a 60-year old. Apparently, in some cases, women don't object to dying of lung cancer...they just don't like being buried wrinkled! Hence, this cosmetic twist may serve as an effective motivation.

We hope we've made the point that more and more evidence is accumulating to confirm the dangers of tobacco. Apparently, this information hasn't reached or isn't being taken seriously by our youngsters.

Did you know:
- one out of every eight 12-14 year old kids smoke?
- 30% of American high-school seniors smoke every day
- The United States Public Health Service says that among teen-age girls, a cigarette smoker is much more likely than a non-

smoker to use marijuana, get drunk, engage in sex, and hate school.

In the light of these extraordinary nontrivia regarding America's youth, you might want to check this questionnaire.

This self-test prepared by the Office on Smoking and Health, is designed to help teenagers understand their feelings about cigarette smoking. Included are statements that some youngsters have made about cigarette smoking and cigarette smokers. We acknowledge permission to reprint this form. After reading each statement, insert a 3 if you agree, if you neither agree or disagree put a 2, should you disagree place a 1 in the appropriate box.

1. Even though lung cancer and heart disease can be caused by other things, smoking cigarettes is still a significant factor in those diseases.

2. Cigarette smoking can harm the health of teenagers.

3. Even if cigarettes don't kill you, they can cut down on what you might get out of life.

4. I believe the health information about smoking is true.

5. There's nothing wrong with smoking cigarettes as long as you don't smoke too many.

Now total your first five answers and put your grade in this box.

Scores on this set of statements tell how much you know or believe about the effects of cigarette smoking on health.

The average teenager scores 12, which indicates a high level of belief in the health hazards of smoking. If you scored 13 or above, you're well aware of the harmful effects of smoking and likely are concerned.

If your grade is between 9 and 12, you show concern about the health risks, but slightly less than the average young person. A total of less than 9 signifies you have little knowledge of smoking dangers or you've not thought enough about them to have formed a strong opinion.

There's another way of looking at this issue.

6. Cigarette smoke smells bad.

7. Cigarette smokers should be kept apart from nonsmokers in public places.

8. I prefer the company of girls/boys who don't smoke.

9. Cigarette smoking should be forbidden inside public places.

10. If I smoke around other people, I take away their right to breathe clean air.

Once again, put your total for these five questions in the space:

There's a growing feeling that people who don't

smoke have the right to breathe clean nicotine-free air. Your score on this series of questions indicates how sensitive you are to how other people feel about breathing cigarette smoke. The average score for all teenagers is 10; 12's considered a high score—indicating a person who would rather not be around smokers and would like to see them kept apart from others in public places. If you scored below 6, you apparently don't feel that cigarette smoke bothers nonsmokers.

Now how do you think you feel about the positive effects of smoking?

11. People smoke cigarettes to help them think more clearly.

12. Smoking cigarettes can help you enjoy life more.

13. People who smoke seem to be more at ease with others.

14. Smoking cigarettes gives you a good feeling.

15. Smoking cigarettes seems to make good times even better.

This set of questions looks at what people believe they get out of smoking a cigarette.

In the event, your grade is 12 or above, you believe that people benefit a great deal from smoking. The average teenager scores 7, which indicates that most young people don't believe cigarettes contribute much to a person's enjoyment of life. A total of 6 or below shows that you don't see many positive virtues to smoking cigarettes.

Finally, let's check the rationalizations.

16. It's okay for teenagers to experiment with cigarettes if they quit before it becomes a habit. ☐

17. Cigarette smoking is harmful only if a person inhales. ☐

18. There is no danger in smoking cigars or pipes. ☐

19. Cigarettes low in tar and nicotine can't harm your health. ☐

20. Teenagers who smoke regularly can quit for good any time they like. ☐

☐

Would you believe your excuse score?

Most youngsters who smoke, although they believe that smoking is harmful to health, can find reasons for ignoring this fact. They manufacture justifications for overlooking the dangers of smoking, or pretend there are circumstances where there are no hazards in smoking. A high total, 12 or above, says "It can't happen to me," or "Here are the reasons it's all right for me to smoke now." On the other hand, though, a low mark, 6 or below, indicates that you aren't trying to pretend that it's all right to smoke.

The average score of all teenagers is only 7, indicating that most young people don't try to explain away the disadvantages of smoking. This is true for smokers and nonsmokers alike!

There is another excellent questionnaire designed to evaluate teenage social awareness and self-understanding which isn't being incorporated here for space reasons. However, more information can be obtained in the bibliography (p. 289).

You may wish to know that there are many agencies who are interested in helping smokers quit. Several are listed below.

- Action on Smoking and Health (ASH) provides a wide range of news related to smoking and supports the efforts to assist the rights of nonsmokers in medical, legal, regulatory, commercial, institutional, and even humorous dimensions. They may be contacted at 2013 H Street, N.W., Washington, D.C. 20006. The telephone number is 202/659-4310.
- The American Cancer Society, 4 West 35th Street, New York, New York 10001, (212/736-3030), publishes a quarterly newsletter. There are approximately 2000 local chapters. A number of them offer smoking cessation programs and clinics. Full particulars can usually be obtained through a local chapter.
- The Office on Smoking and Health, U.S. Department of Health and Human Services, Technical Information Center, Park Building Room 1-16, 5600 Fishers Lane, Rockville, Maryland 20857, (301/443-1690). They publish a number of information bulletins in the field of smoking.

Additional information on smoking in the workplace is available in Chapter 10.

And finally, much valuable information can be found in the forthcoming resource section of this chapter.

RESOURCES

1. Cheraskin, E., Ringsdorf, W. M. Jr., and

Medford, F. H.
Eating Habits of Smokers and Nonsmokers
The Journal of the International Academy of Preventive Medicine 2: #2, 9-17, Second Quarter 1975.

Dietary intake and daily tobacco consumption were assessed in approximately 700 members of the health professions. It was found that, although the diets of both smokers and nonsmokers contained about the same number of calories, there was a great difference in the proportions of nutrients. On a mean basis, for the smoker group, the intake of almost every vitamin, mineral and amino acid studied was less than for the nonsmoker group. Many of the differences were statistically significant. Interestingly enough, the smokers consume a statistically significantly greater amount of refined carbohydrates.

2. Daniell, H. W.
Smoker's Wrinkles: A Study in the Epidemiology of "Crow's Feet"
Annals of Internal Medicine 75: #6, 873-880, December 1971.

A relatively simple method of assessing the severity of facial skin wrinkles is described. The technique can be rapidly learned and easily used by untrained persons. In a study of 1104 subjects, the severity of wrinkling correlated with a history of habitual cigarette smoking, after adjustment for age and outdoor exposure. The relationship between cigarette smoking and wrinkling was striking in both sexes soon after the age of 30, was related to the duration and intensity of cigarette smoking, and was clearly more pronounced than was the association between wrinkling and admitted outdoor exposure. Smokers in the 40- to 49-year age group were as likely to be prominently wrinkled as nonsmokers who were 20 years older.

3. Eysenck, H. J.
   The Causes and Effects of Smoking
   1980. Beverly Hills, Sage Publications.

   Professor Eysenck of the Institute of Psychiatry at the University of London reviews the overall problem of smoking. What's especially unique in this book and relevant to this chapter is the awareness that there's been relatively little work done on the fate of giving up smoking. Additionally, scant attention has been accorded the study of personality traits of those who surrender the habit, as compared with continued smokers, nonsmokers, and people who tried to give up but failed. Included in his book are several interesting and unique questionnaires. First is the Eysenck Personality Questionnaire which scores personality traits. The second relates to changes following cessation of smoking. The third inquires about occasions for smoking.

4. Fielding, J. E.
   Smoking: Health Effects and Control (First of Two Parts)

New England Journal of Medicine 313: #8, 491-498, 22 August 1985.

Cigarette smoking has been identified as the single most important source of preventable morbidity and premature mortality in each of the reports of the United States Surgeon General produced since 1964. It's been estimated that an average of 5 1/2 minutes of life is lost for each cigarette smoked. This means a net reduction in life expectancy of five to eight years. The economic burden on each nonsmoker for providing medical care for smoking-induced illness exceeds $100, paid primarily through taxes and health insurance premiums. Smoking, incidentally, is responsible for 25% of all the mortality caused by fire and accounts for close to 500 million dollars in other losses.

5. Greenhalgh, R. M.
Smoking and Arterial Disease
1981. Melbourne, Pitman Medical

In this excellent book, evidence that arterial disease of all types may be precipitated by cigarette smoking is examined and discussed. In the early chapters it's clearly established that there's a connection between smoking and peripheral arterial, cerebrovascular, coronary heart, and aneurysmal diseases. The fact that people in general wish to stop smoking was clearly shown in October 1977 during a television program in which was included a 10-minute feature on smoke-ending with an offer of help; a free anti-smoking kit for those who cared to phone or write in. The response was staggering. Six-hundred thousand people asked for the kit. Clearly, many of the smokers who want to stop smoking feel they need help; that is, they feel too dependent to do it by themselves.

6. Marlett, G. A. and Gordon, J. R.
Relapse Prevention
1985. New York, The Guilford Press.

Relapse Prevention (RP) is a generic designation that refers to a wide range of strategies designed to prevent relapse in the area of addictive behavior change. The primary focus of RP is on the crucial issue of maintenance in the habit-change process. The purpose is twofold: to prevent the occurrence of initial lapses after one has embarked on a program of habit-change, and/or to prevent any lapse from escalating into a total relapse. Although the RP model has general implications for habit-change with a variety of target behaviors, the main emphasis in this particular book is on addictive behaviors including problem drinking, substance use, eating disorders, compulsive gambling, and smoking. Special mention should be made to Chapter 8, by Saul Shiffman, which deals with Preventing Relapse in Ex-smokers: A Self-Management Approach.

7. Medical News
New Knowledge About Nicotine Effects
Journal of the American Medical Association 247: #17, 2333-2338, 7 May 1982.

Remember the cigarette advertisements of the 1940s: "Reach for a Lucky instead of a sweet" and "Have a Camel with your meal and after it—they satisfy"? Recent research suggests that such advertisements were indeed accurate. There's evidence that cigarettes may reduce the desire for sweets and help some people achieve greater satisfaction from their meals. And the critical ingredient seems to be nicotine. In fact, a wealth of recent information suggests that nicotine in cigarettes is responsible for a host of physiologic and psychologic effects and that these metabolic alterations and mood changes represent a major reason why people smoke—and also why they find it so hard to stop smoking.

8. Morgan, G. L. and Golding, J. F.
The Psychopharmacology of Smoking
1984. Cambridge, Cambridge University Press

This book discusses the overall problem of smoking. However, of particular interest is the third part which attempts to evaluate the various health education programs, interventions and termination strategies assayed over the past twenty years. These strategies can be divided further into those of a general nature such as mass communication of antismoking propaganda and those of a very precise type such as problems involving small groups or individual smokers. There's an excellent summary of all of the current methods used in the treatment of the smoking habit.

9. Office on Smoking and Health
   1980 Directory: On-Going Research in Smoking and Health
   1980. United States Department of Health and Human Services.

   This is the eighth edition of the Directory of On-Going Research in Smoking and Health. It's a compilation of current research conducted throughout the world on smoking, tobacco and tobacco use. What's particularly relevant here is the increasing interest in the areas of behavioral and educational research. This trend to study why people smoke and how to influence smoking behavior documents the interest of the medical community in ascertaining approaches to reduce morbidity and mortality attributed to smoking. The directory summarizes 1129 projects from 42 countries. The United States contributed 649 of them.

10. Office on Smoking and Health
    Teenage Cigarette Smoking Self-Test
    PHS 82-50189 United States Department of Health and Human Services

    Teenagers need to take the time to become informed in order to make a thoughtful decision about smoking. The self-test allows the young person to explore his or her own knowledge of the health effects of smoking, feelings about smokers, and views on why people begin smoking. The first part of this test form is cited in the body of this chapter and deals with the teenager's knowledge of smoking. A second portion designed to analyze social awareness and self-understanding is not included here but can be obtained from the Office on Smoking and Health, Rockville, Maryland 20857 (use the PHS publication number listed above).

11. Report of the Surgeon-General
The Health Consequences of Smoking: Chronic Obstructive Lung Disease
1984. Washington, D. C., United States Department of Health and Human Services.

Smokers can realize a substantial health benefit from quitting smoking, no matter how long they have smoked. As this report clearly states, sufficient evidence now exists to document lung function improvement in smokers who have quit. Ex-smokers can look forward to improved future health, avoiding long-term and possibly severe disability, or even death from chronic obstructive lung disease. Of particular relevance are the two chapters in this report which summarize research studies using two vastly different cessation approaches. One focuses on the role of physicians in assisting patient populations to quit smoking. The other looks at community-wide intervention programs. Both have been shown to exert a significant impact on reducing the number of smokers in the American population.

12. Sandler, D. P., Wilcox, A. J., and Everson, R. B.
Cumulative Effects of Lifetime Passive Smoking on Cancer Risk

Lancet 1: #8424, 312-315, 9 February 1985.

Cancer risk from cumulative household exposure to cigarette smoke has been evaluated in a case-control study. The overall cancer risk rose steadily and significantly with each additional household member who smoked over an individual's lifetime. Cancer risk was also greater for persons with exposures during both childhood and adulthood than for individuals with exposures during only one period. These trends were observed for both smoking-related and other sites. These preliminary findings suggest that the effects of exposure to the cigarette smoking of others may be greater than has been previously suspected.

16

ARE YOU DRINKING TOO MUCH (ALCOHOL)?

Guess...how many people in America drink booze? According to our best estimate, 3 out of 4 (and believe it or not this is equally true of teenagers) use alcohol. Half guzzle beer. Incidentally, there are only two countries on this planet (the Soviet Union and Poland) which report greater alcohol consumption than in these United States.

What does this mean in terms of well-being? According to the U. S. Department of Health and Human Services, alcohol plays a role in:

- 37 of every 100 suicides

- 50% of all highway accidents
- approximately 7 out of 10 murders
- half of all arrests
- more mental-hospital admissions than for any other single cause

What about the economics? The National Institute on Alcohol Abuse and Alcoholism estimates:
- $10 billion in lost work time per annum
- $2 billion for the health and welfare of alcoholics and their families per year
- $3 billion in property damage, medical expense, insurance costs and the like, yearly
- so this amounts to a total $15 billion drain on the economy annually...or $60 for every man, woman and child in America.

What else makes alcoholism **really** unique?

It's the only well-defined medical syndrome which traditional medicine has been delighted to surrender to a nonmedical group, Alcoholics Anonymous (AA), for care! The record shows that 1 out of 10 patients are actually recommended to AA by their family physician.

The most fascinating piece of nontrivia is:
- The heavy drinker is a man, separated from his wife but not divorced. He's mostly a beer drinker, and he has no religious affiliation.
- The American least likely to have a drinking problem is a woman. She's Jewish, over 50 years old, has a graduate degree, and lives in the rural south.

As one might expect, there are stacks of excellent tests designed to assess drinking habits (for more particulars, check the resources at the end of this chapter). The simplest is the CAGE Quiz which poses four clinical interview questions (see Resource #4 on p. 305). CAGE is an acronym which represents the

first letter in one of the words in each of the four questions. They are:
1. Have you ever felt you ought to CUT down on your drinking?
2. Have people ANNOYED you by critizing your drinking?
3. Have you ever felt bad or GUILTY about your drinking?
4. Have you ever had a drink first thing in the morning to steady your nerves or get rid of a hangover—(EYEOPENER)?

As we've indicated earlier, this is the simplest of the questionnaires and in some circles it's believed to be an adequate detection device. Since its introduction in 1970, CAGE has become recognized as one of the most efficient and effective screening tools. Two or three affirmative answers should create a high index of suspicion. Four positive responses is viewed as sure-fire evidence of alcoholism. Because the CAGE is easy to administer, reliable in identifying alcoholics, and less intimidating than some of the other instruments, it's an appealing first step in detecting the problems.

But it has shortcomings. One of the obvious needs not met by this yay-or-nay questionnaire is the inability to discriminate the **shades of gray** of alcoholism.

To obviate some of the objections to CAGE, a device found to be useful in identifying alcohol dependence is the Michigan Alcoholism Screening Test (MAST). This was developed in 1971 and consists of a series of yes/no questions extracted from the medical literature and found by previous investigators to correlate with alcohol abuse. The original twenty-five questions have been reduced to twenty-four. This form is cited here and we thank Doctor James S. Powers. Also, permission is granted by Southern Medical Journal (77: #7, 852-856, July 1984). Incidentally, there are other thirteen, ten, and thirty-four question versions of the test. It's been administered to more than 7,000 patients and is remarkably specific and sensitive with a less than ten percent false negative rate and high validity in specifying alcoholism.

Try it!

	yes	no
1. Does your wife, husband, a parent, or other near relative ever worry or complain about your drinking?	☐	☐
2. Do you ever feel guilty about your drinking?	☐	☐
3. Have you ever gotten into physical fights when drinking?	☐	☐
4. Do you drink before noon fairly often?	☐	☐

Now score yourself.

Give yourself 1 point for each question you answered in the affirmative. Place your total in the box below:

☐

Now to the next set of questions.

5. Do you feel you are a normal drinker? (By normal we mean you drink less than or as much as most other people.)	☐	☐

6. Have you ever awakened the morn-

		yes	no
	ing after some drinking the night before and found that you could not remember a part of the evening?	☐	☐
7.	Can you stop drinking without a struggle after one or two drinks?	☐	☐
8.	Do friends or relatives think you are a normal drinker?	☐	☐
9.	Are you able to stop drinking when you want to?	☐	☐
10.	Has drinking ever created problems between you and your wife, husband, a parent, or other relative?	☐	☐
11.	Has your wife, husband, a parent, or other near relative ever gone to anyone for help about your drinking?	☐	☐
12.	Have you ever lost boy/girl friends because of your drinking?	☐	☐
13.	Have you ever gotten into trouble at work because of your drinking?	☐	☐
14.	Have you ever lost a job because of drinking?	☐	☐
15.	Have you ever neglected your obligations, your family, or your work for two or more days in a row because you were drinking?	☐	☐

	yes	no
16. Have you ever been told you have liver trouble? Cirrhosis?	☐	☐
17. After heavy drinking have you ever had delirium tremens (DTs) or severe shaking or heard voices or seen things that weren't really there?	☐	☐
18. Have you ever been a patient in a psychiatric hospital or on a psychiatric ward of a general hospital where drinking was part of the problem that resulted in hospitalization?	☐	☐
19. Have you ever been seen at a psychiatric or mental health clinic or gone to any doctor, social worker, or clergyman for help with any emotional problem, where drinking was part of the problem?	☐	☐
20. Have you ever been arrested for drunken driving under the influence of alcoholic beverages?	☐	☐
21. Have you ever been arrested, even for a few hours, because of other drunken behavior?	☐	☐

For each of these questions 5 through 21, which were answered **yes**, give yourself a 2. Insert the total in the box provided:

☐

	yes	no

Now for the final three questions.

22. Have you ever attended a meeting of Alcoholics Anonymous? ☐ ☐

23. Have you ever gone to anyone for help about your drinking? ☐ ☐

24. Have you ever been in a hospital because of drinking? ☐ ☐

Finally, for these last three querries, give yourself a 5 for each yes response and insert the total in the appropriate box:

☐

Now we're ready to find what your overall grade is:

Score for questions: ☐ + ☐ + ☐ = ☐
1-4   5-21   22-24   total

Let's analyze your score:

Should your overall mark be 0 to 4—you're definitely nonalcoholic.

With a grade of 5 or 6—there's a small possibility of alcoholism.

However, if your total was 7 or more—there's strong evidence of disease.

Finally, positive responses to questions 22, 23 and 24 are virtually diagnostic of the problem.

Let's assume that your score suggests a problem. What are the possible causes and what to do about it?

For the moment, the concensus is that alcoholism is a psychosocial problem that can be resolved by means of psychosocial treatment. This is certainly part and parcel of the tenets of Alcoholics Anonymous as well as the customary approach by psychiatrists, psychologists, social workers and the clergy.

In more recent times, greater attention is being directed to other lifestyle conditions as a major contributor to alcoholism.

And so, is alcoholism really just a **social** disease?

Call an ex-alcoholic **reformed** at your own risk. No moral issue has been resolved when a drinker has been cured of his disease.

Mercedes McCambridge is one of many well-known personalities who is an **out-of-the-closet** former alcoholic pleading for better public understanding of America's number one drug addiction—and least understood ailment. Her message, a simple one, is delivered with all the fire and guts she can muster: "alcoholics aren't evil, weak willed, or immoral. I know, because I've been one. Alcoholism isn't a 'social' disease. It's some kind of disaster."

But what kind? While many authorities now agree that there's no single cause for habitual drinking, emphasis has most often been placed on family relationships. If there has been mental illness in the family background—or criminality, neurosis, serious parental discord, divorce, or alcoholism, your chances of becoming an alcoholic multiply.

One theory suggests that people who come from unstable backgrounds turn to the bottle in time of need, while those with solid, supportive families look to friends and relatives. But there are investigators who challenge this flight-from-reality hypothesis which has been given such a wide arena in which to spar with supposedly villainous parents.

Put another way, alcoholism does indeed seem to run in families. Hence, there's no question that, to a varying degree, there's **familial** implications. However, the mere fact that something runs in the family doesn't necessarily mean that it's genetic. This brings us back to the nature versus nurture debate referred to in Chapter 14 on diet. There's now evidence that the familial inclination for alcohol may also be an environmental issue.

A great many researchers who have lifted the alcoholic off the couch and placed him under the scrutiny of a microscope are convinced that uncontrolled drinking is a metabolic disorder that can be treated by nutritional therapy.

Doctors are of course, aware of the fact that alcoholics frequently suffer with malnutrition. However, it's usually assumed that poor nutrition is the result of the alcoholism, not a causative factor. In other words, faulty nutrition of the brain cells is simply not viewed as a contributor to alcoholism. Yet, there have now been studies in humans and in lower animals suggesting the importance of diet/nutrition in the genesis of alcoholism.

One of the most intriguing experiments was done at Loma Linda University in California where investigators induced a craving for alcohol in rats by feeding them a diet high in refined-carbohydrate food, low in vitamins, minerals, and proteins. The rats were not psychologically stressed. They were certainly not reared by mean parents but they turned eagerly to drink when provided a typical **teenager's** diet! Lo and behold with retraining the rats to good eating habits, their alcohol problem vanished. The rat studies, to the extent possible, have been validated in humans. For more information regarding these lower animal and people experiments, check the references (#11 and #13) at the end of this chapter.

And don't forget, alcoholism isn't just for grown-

ups. How big a concern is it in the teenager?
- 93% of male and 87% of female high-school seniors have tried booze
- one out of four 12-13 year old boys have a drink a week
- on some campuses, 9 out of 10 students use alcohol
- in fact, the average college student has 400 alcoholic drinks a year...more than one a day!

On the basis of these staggering numbers, is drinking becoming a problem for kids? Why don't you and your youngster(s) check it out. These 12 questions from **A Message to Teenagers** reprinted with permission of Alcoholics Anonymous World Services Inc.

Please mark a yes or no to each of the following:

		yes	no
1.	Do you drink because you have problems? To relax?	☐	☐
2.	Do you drink when you get mad at other people, your friends or parents?	☐	☐
3.	Do you prefer to drink alone, rather than with others?	☐	☐
4.	Are your grades starting to slip? Are you goofing off on your job?	☐	☐
5.	Did you ever try to stop drinking or drink less—and fail?	☐	☐
6.	Have you begun to drink in the morning, before school or work?	☐	☐

		yes	no
7.	Do you gulp your drinks?	☐	☐
8.	Do you ever have loss of memory due to your drinking?	☐	☐
9.	Do you lie about your drinking?	☐	☐
10.	Do you ever get into trouble when you are drinking?	☐	☐
11.	Do you get drunk when you drink, even when you don't mean to?	☐	☐
12.	Do you think it's cool to be able to hold your liquor?	☐	☐

If you can answer yes to any **one** of these questions, maybe it's time you took a serious look at what your drinking might be doing to you.

It's obvious that there are lots of questionnaires to help us decide whether we are alcoholic or threatening to become a problem case.

The next and last issue is to decide what to do about it.

The point should be reemphasized that Alcoholics Anonymous represents the single and most classical avenue to first look into for people with the drinking syndrome. You might wish to check with your local chapter for more particulars.

Finally, it would be well to recall the story of the rats and their interest in alcoholism resulting from experimental dietary manipulation. A good place to begin is by examining your own eating habits made possible by reviewing Chapter 14. However, other lifestyle characteristics may contribute to alcoholism and its solutions (such as physical activity).

For more particulars, consult the resource list attached to this chapter. You'll find interesting and practical descriptions and answers to the prevention and treatment of this devastating disorder!

RESOURCES

1. Cheraskin, E. and Ringsdorf, W. M., Jr.
   New Hope for Incurable Diseases
   1971. New York, Exposition Press (hardback)
   1973. New York, Arco Publishing Company (paperback)

   This book contains a fairly extensive chapter on alcoholism including an interesting bibliographic section. The thrust is that there's a large dietary/nutritional component in the etiology of this syndrome. Very simply, there is much evidence suggesting that hypoglycemia might well be a significant contributor to alcoholism. This is emphasized in Chapter 7.

2. Cheraskin, E., Ringsdorf, W. M., Jr. and Brecher, A.
   Psychodietetics
   1974. New York, Stein and Day (hardback)
   1976. New York, Bantam Books, Inc. (paperback)

   This book is designed for lay-educational purposes to analyze the food-and-mood connection. One section (chapter 4) summarizes the importance of diet in alcoholism. There's a fairly extensive bibliography which shows clearly that diet/nutrition plays an important role in this heretofore social syndrome.

3. Eckardt, M. J., Harford, T. C., Kaelber, C. T., Parker, E. S., Rosenthal, L. S., Ryback, R. S., Salmoiraghi, G. C., Vanderveen, E. and Warren, K. R.
Health Hazards Associated With Alcohol Consumption
Journal of the American Medical Association 246: #8, 648-666, 7 August 1981.

This excellent review first discusses the pharmacologic properties of ethanol to establish it as a drug, and then deals with alcohol-drug interactions. Certain nondisease health risks that might require medical treatment have also been examined and tabulated including alcohol-related suicides, accidents, and criminal behavior. The overall organization used in this report is to define each health hazard, to establish its relationship to alcohol use, including mechanism whenever possible, and to provide estimates of the extent of alcohol involvement.

4. Ewing, J. A.
Detecting Alcoholism: The CAGE Questionnaire
Journal of the American Medical Association 252: #14, 1905-1907, 12 October 1984.

The CAGE questions were developed from a

clinical study undertaken in 1968 at North Carolina Memorial Hospital. This particular questionnaire has become recognized as one of the most efficient and effective screening devices. Two or three affirmative answers should create a high index of suspicion. Four positive responses is viewed as definite alcoholism. The CAGE is seen not only as easy to administer and reliable in distinguishing alcoholics but also as less intimidating than some of the other instruments.

5. Favazza, A. R. and Pires, J.
The Michigan Alcoholism Screening Test: Application in a General Military Hospital
Quarterly Journal of Studies on Alcohol 35: #3, 925-929, September 1974.

In 1971, the Michigan Alcoholism Screening Test (MAST) was reported by Selzer to be a valid and simple instrument for the identification of alcoholism. Scores on this same test given to active-duty Navy enlisted men at the U. S. Naval Hospital in Oakland, California, indicated alcoholism in 97% of diagnosed alcoholics. This certainly confirms the utility of this simple and quick instrument.

6. Horrobin, D. F.
Alcohol—Blessing and Curse of Mankind!
Executive Health 17: #9, June 1981.

If you choose people on the street at random, eliminate those who have obvious problems with alcohol, and screen the rest for alcoholic liver damage, 15 to 25 percent of these seemingly normal people who all believe their alcohol consumption is safely under control will have evidence of liver damage due to too much alcohol! The prevention and treatment of alcohol must be directed to two ends. Craving for alcohol must be reduced and the physical damage which can occur for lack of certain prostaglandins (PGs) must be avoided or reversed. This excellent report analyzes the options available.

7. Kolonel, L. N. and Lee, J.
Husband-wife correspondence in smoking, drinking and dietary habits
American Journal of Clinical Nutrition 34: 99-104, January 1981.

In order to determine the extent of correlation between husbands and wives in their personal habits, a sample of 281 spouse pairs was interviewed concerning their drinking as well as their smoking and eating habits. The correspondence for wine was significant and less so for beer. There was good relationship between husbands and wives for a majority of the food items, the exceptions being foods that are more likely to be eaten away from home.

8. Medical News
High Carbohydrate Diet Affects Rat's Alcohol Intake
Journal of the American Medical Association 212: #6, 976, 11 May 1970.

The experiment reported in this chapter as Reference #11 was originally presented at the annual Federation of the American Society of Experimental Biology in 1970. It underlined, in lower animal studies, the effects of diet in general and vitamins/minerals in particular, as it promotes and discourages alcohol dependency.

9. Null, G. and Null, S.
    Alcohol and Nutrition
    1976. New York, Pyramid

This paper back, designed for lay educational purposes, discusses the overall problems in civilized societies. Of particular relevance to this chapter is the emphasis placed upon the biologic rather than the psychosocial factors which contribute to this syndrome. Considerable attention is devoted to the not-so-often-discussed role of diet/nutrition in alcoholism.

10. Powers, J. S. and Spickard, A.
    Michigan Alcoholism Screening Test to Diagnose Early Alcoholism in a General Practice.
    Southern Medical Journal 77: #7, 852-856, July 1984.

General medical patients can be easily screened for alcohol dependence on a routine basis. The Michigan Alcoholism Screening Test (MAST) is a 24-item yes/no questionnaire concerning alcohol-related behavior. When it was included in the history self-administered to new patients in an internal medicine out-patient service, it uncovered unsuspected alcohol dependence. All patients with significant MAST scores had complaints related to active drinking.

11. Register, U. D., Marsh, S. R., Thurston, C. T., Fields, B. J., Horning, M. C., Hardinge, M.D., and Sanchez, A.
Influence of Nutrients on Intake of Alcohol.
Journal of the American Dietetic Association 61: #2, 159-162, August 1972.

This study was conducted to determine whether a teenage-type diet, known to be marginal in nutrients, would elicit drinking behavior in rats similar to that induced by purified diets deficient in nutrients. In addition to the marginal nutritional content, dietary items, such as coffee and spices, were also studied. It was observed that rats fed the control human diet maintained a low level of alcohol intake. However, animals provided a marginal teenage-diet continued to increase their alcohol consumption throughout the study. Groups fed diets supplemented with either coffee or caffeine consumed significantly larger quantities of alcohol as compared with animals fed the unsupplemented diet. Conversely, the group given the marginal teenage-diet supplemented with vitamins had a significantly lower alcohol intake. When heavy drinkers on the teenage-diets were fed the controlled diet, alcohol consumption was significantly decreased. These data suggest the possibility that metabolic controls to drinking exist which are sensitive to dietary factors. This is a must for those interested in carefully controlled alcohol studies in lower animals.

12. Williams R. J.
Alcoholism: The Nutritional Approach
1959. Austin, University of Texas Press

This world famous investigator, who has devoted years of studying the problem of alcoholism, believes that it's a physical and usually a curable disease. While recognizing that psychiatry, medicine, and religion, as well as nutrition, must all play a part in the rehabilitation of the alcoholic, he asserts that unless the body chemistry is so adjusted that the appetite mechanisms function properly, nothing can bring success. The best hope in the fight against alcoholism, then, continues to be its prevention through dietary controls. In this valuable and highly recommended book, he presents his views in layman's language.

13. Williams R. J.
The Prevention of Alcoholism Through Nutrition
1981. New York, Bantam Books.

It would be difficult for anyone other than Dr. Williams to approach the subject of preventing alcoholism through nutrition with authority. He is the discoverer of some of the important vitamins which are essential to alcohol metabolism, and wrote the only published book dealing with biochemical individuality, the vital basis upon which the existence of the disease, alcoholism, rests. Dr. Williams offers seven simple steps that can prevent alcoholism, and thoroughly explores the connection between alcoholism and heredity; high risk individuals; the insidious relationship between appetite and alcohol; and why young people are more susceptible to alcohol addiction.

17

HOW ACTIVE ARE YOU?

The importance of activity to well-being and sickness is unquestioned. If you don't believe it, tape your good arm to your body. In a matter of weeks it'll shrivel. This highly predictable demonstration, with scads of supporting data, underlines the importance of motion to every cell, tissue, organ, and site. If you're the kind who wants more proof, one month of bedrest can cause a bone loss of approximately four percent. This in turn may contribute to brittle bones and dowager's hump. In other words, it confirms the old adage, "if you don't use it, you'll lose it!"

Now, couple this with the obvious changes in physical activity which parallels our modern mechanization. In the old days—Dad played with the kids on Sunday. Now Pop sits in front of the boob tube with a six-pack of beer and pretzels during the Sunday afternoon football marathon.

And add to this, there's increasing evidence of the possible cause-and-effect connections between physical inactivity and many diverse and seemingly not associated with exercise diseases. (For example, did you know that one can reduce the blood sugar of a diabetic 50 to 80 milligrams percent by simply walking one half mile in 12 minutes?)

So, obviously, exercise has its benefits.

In a recent survey, people who are regular exercisers were asked why they do it. Here's what they said:

- 8 out of 10 reported a general feeling of improvement
- half said it was relaxing
- 50% reported sounder sleep
- 4 out of 10 felt they were more alert, made them look better
- 1/3 reported better mental concentration
- about the same number claimed better self-discipline and improved self-image
- 1 out of 3 insist that they can better cope with pressure
- 25% noted increased assertiveness and creativity
- 1 out of 5 acknowledged better sex life
- Finally, 10% even claimed exercise helped reduce tobacco consumption

And if you need more trivia...Democrats jog more than Republicans...Catholics more likely than Protestants...and single twice as likely as married people.

To add to the confusion out there in the real world, **physical activity** and **exercise** may or may not mean the same. To the literati, physical activity suggests all movement; exercise usually implies organized and generally more strenuous action. In other words, all exercise involves physical movement. However, all physical motion need not necessarily be synonymous with what we envisage as exercise. For example, taking a walk isn't generally viewed as an exercise experience. Put simply, unlike exercise, physical activity like breathing is indispensable.

So what's the problem? What excuses do we hear?

- 43 out of every 100 people tell us they don't have time to exercise
- 16 seem not to have the willpower
- 12% just don't feel like it
- 9 will give you a medical reason
- 8 tell you they just lack energy
- and 12 cook up some other excuse

For our purposes here, the immediate need is to establish the role of physical activity as one possible solution to our many different problems. Next, it would be helpful to ascertain our own level of physical motion.

As one might expect, there are many available questionnaires. Obviously, some are complex. A very simple one is a four-question form cited here. Reproduced by permission from Wayne A. Payne, Ed.D. and Dale B. Hahn, Ph.D. **Understanding Your Health** and St. Louis, 1986, Times Mirror/Mosby College Publishing

Try it.

Grade yourself according to your participation.

1. How frequently do you engage in some type of individual or group fitness activity?

a. less than once a week (1 point)
   b. once or twice a week (2 points)
   c. three times a week (3 points)
   d. four or five times a week (4 points)
   e. more than five times a week (5 points) ☐

2. When participating in these fitness activities, what is the duration of your participation?

   a. less than 5 minutes (1 point)
   b. between 5 and 15 minutes (2 points)
   c. approximately 20 minutes (3 points)
   d. between 20 and 30 minutes (4 points)
   e. more than 30 minutes (5 points) ☐

3. How would you classify the intensity of your participation in fitness activities?

   a. very low level (1 point)
   b. low level (2 points)
   c. moderate level (3 points)
   d. high level (4 points)
   e. very high level (5 points) ☐

4. How frequently are your fitness activities continuous and enjoyable?

   a. never (1 point)
   b. occasionally (2 points)
   c. half of time (3 points)
   d. frequently (4 points)
   e. all the time (5 points) ☐

Now add up your total points and insert your score in the box below:

☐

If your score is 16 to 20, then your physical activity program is very likely to be providing you with an excellent conditioning effect. This is another way of saying that you're involved in a great schedule. On the other hand, a score of 13 to 15 suggests adequate but not superlative effort. An overall grade of 7 to 12, signals an inadequate program. A score of 4 to 6, isn't good.

Mention has been made earlier in this chapter (and in other sections) that there are all kinds of questionnaires. Some are simple, some complex; many short and others long; sometimes sophisticated, some nonspecific. Here's one that smacks of uniqueness. It's specialness lays in the fact that it plays on **vanity**. You may remember the quasi-humorous point made (Chapter 15) that women apparently do not object to dying of cancer; they just don't like being buried wrinkled! The point of that story, and it's also germane here, is that vanity may play a significant diagnostic (as well as motivational) role.

So, take this questionnaire by Millie Cooper of Aerobics fame. We thank her along with her publisher, Bantam Books, for allowing us the use of this form.

Here are ten questions obviously more suited for the female though many applicable to men, to help you discover what your reasons might be for wanting to start an activity program. Check the appropriate box.

		yes	no
1.	I'm satisfied with my weight.	☐	☐
2.	My weight doesn't fluctuate much.	☐	☐

3. I'm pleased with my body's con-

	yes	no
tours.	☐	☐
4. I'm happy about my dress size.	☐	☐
5. My family and friends give me sincere compliments on my appearance.	☐	☐
6. I admire my figure clad in a swimsuit.	☐	☐
7. I haven't found flab or cellulite anywhere on my body.	☐	☐
8. Stress doesn't increase my appetite.	☐	☐
9. I don't have a strong desire to look like someone else.	☐	☐
10. I characterize myself nutrition-and-health conscious, moderate in all my habits.	☐	☐

If you checked **no** to any of these questions you have one more reason for embarking on an organized activity plan.

What are the solutions? Fortunately, there are many including running, cycling, swimming, and competitive sports (e.g. tennis, racquetball, handball, etc.). And lucky for us, the state of the art today makes it possible to actually measure our needs. In other words, we now have in hand the knowledge to write, as-it-were a physical activity prescription stating how many minutes and how hard one needs to run or swim or play tennis.

The most comprehensive and yet simple prescriptions have been written by Kenneth H. Cooper, M.D. and described in great detail in a number of his publications summarized as suggested readings at the end of this chapter.

It's well to point out that Doctor Cooper has painstakingly examined the various forms of activity. Additionally, he's reduced them to measurable amounts so that anyone can pick and choose among them and know how much exercise is necessary to produce a beneficial effect. His conclusions are based on observations that all popular exercises have been more-or-less scientifically measured for the amount of energy it costs the body to perform them. These amounts have been translated into points—the more energy it costs, the more points; less energy, less points—and the number of points necessary to produce an optimum level of fitness, within limits, has been established. The purpose of his program is to earn a basic minimum every week, by whatever combination of exercises you choose.

Doctor Cooper has put his ideas into an acronym FIT which represents **f**requency, **i**ntensity, and **t**ime. (This formula is utilized in the first questionnaire beginning on p. 315).

Frequency suggests how often you should exercise. In general, he prefers that there be three or four sessions per week.

Intensity refers to the vigorousness of the sessions. The general rule is that you should be moving at a brisk enough pace to notice a definite increase in your breathing and pulse rate and eventually begin to perspire. It's important to understand that one shouldn't be panting so hard that you can't talk.

That's overdoing it.

Time refers to how long each session lasts.

Obviously, the recommendations vary with the initial health state, the age and sex of the individual, the type of exercise deemed most practical and pleasurable. For example, running 2 miles at a 10-minute mile pace, 4 times a week, with the heart rate 140+ for 20 minutes is an average adequate prescription for most people. The recommendations should not be rigid. For instance, the same benefits can be derived by aerobic dancing for 30 minutes, 3 times a week, with the heart rate 130+ for 30 minutes.

For more particulars to satisfy the needs of different persons for varied exercise programs, check the resources.

The good news is that aerobic programs are now available to accomodate the needs of just about everybody.

The not-so-good-news is, if you stop and think about it, there's an element of illogic. Picture this, there's the implication that one can sit immobilized for 23 1/2 hours a day as long as one then runs for 30 minutes in one's underwear at the crack of dawn!

The simple fact of the matter is that there's really only one truly physiologic activity program. **Walking is the only exercise in common sense!** Just about every other discipline suggests the element of artificiality, uncomfortableness, and in some cases even danger.

What's so great about walking?
- It's easy to learn. In fact, you don't have to take lessons to do it.
- It's available for the rest of your life. When you're older you don't have to scale down to a less exhausting program.
- You can set your own schedule. You might like

to walk in the morning before going to work or walk to and from your job or make it an evening stroll.
- You can do it alone or with someone else and enjoy conversation. (Remember, the family that walks together talks together.)
- It's certainly the least strenuous of all forms of exercise. While there are many happy runners, it's rare to find a runner happy running (just look at their faces).
- And, would you believe, one survey found the drop-out rate (25%) in the walking program. On the other hand, three out of four high intensity exercisers, like runners, quit within three to six months.
- It doesn't cost anything. You don't have to pay fees or join a private club to become a walker— all you need do is step outside your door.
- The only equipment required is a sturdy, comfortable pair of shoes. Most walking can be accomplished in street clothes with or without modifications (witness the many ladies walking to work or on their lunch hour dressed for business with their sneakers).
- And a big and positive payoff is that walkers invariably report that they feel better, sleep better and that their mental outlook improves. (A study showed that a 15-minute walk was followed by at least a one-hour tranquility period.) At the University of Florida in Gainesville, a recent study confirmed that only 10% of walkers reported anxiety; one out of two nonexercisers felt anxious.
- It is unchallenged for weight loss and improvement in body composition. At Rockefeller University in New York, experiments suggest

moderate exercise like walking stimulates the flow of adrenalin and endorphins which reduce appetite. They state that you don't work up an appetite with exercise...if anything, you work it down.
- Not to be ignored is that walking is fraught with fewer physical complications. The orthopedist and podiatrist will attest to their booming business with the advent of vigorous exercise. A survey taken showed that 6 out of 10 runners were disabled at least part of the year by injuries. And why not? Joggers land with up to three times their body weight with each step.
- And, let's not forget the actual dangers more often associated with strenuous activity including heart attacks, strokes and even death!
- On a more positive note, walking encourages longevity. (Men who walked nine miles a week were found to have a 21% lower risk of death than those who walked less than three miles.)

If you want more about the wonderful world of walking check the several books listed in the bibliographic section at the end of this chapter.

The greatest counterargument to these reasons for walking is that it seems to lack the desired quantification offered earlier in connection with more strenuous exercise programs. The simple fact of the matter is that one can measure the walking experience just as one can quantify the other programs. Examples may be found in the aerobics literature and listed in the resources.

For the moment, and as one example, here's a five question form which provides some measurable assessment of the walking phenomenon. We wish to thank John W. Farquhar, M.D. for granting us permission to use it.

Check the box that represents your present habits.

my habit

1. brisk walking 5 times per week for 45 minutes each (0 points) ☐

2. brisk walking 3 times per week for 30 minutes each (1 point) ☐

3. brisk walking 2 times per week for 30 minutes each
or
normal walking 4 1/2 to 6 miles daily (2 points) ☐

4. normal walking 2 1/2 to 4 1/2 miles daily (3 points) ☐

5. normal walking less than 2 1/2 miles daily (4 points) ☐

Your possible score could range from 0 to 4. If you are Mr. or Mrs. America your grade will probably be a 2; a super walker would net a 0. Of course, a total of 4 is the worse possible score—it's for sure, you need a change.

Let's exit on these three notes. First, our civilization has clearly moved us into immobility. Second, there's a simple solution...just start putting one foot in front of the other. Finally, the evidence is convincing to suggest that, if and when the same effort is spent studying physical activity in health and sickness as has been expended on penicillin and AZT, there won't be a cell, tissue or organ not favorably influenced by motion.

RESOURCES

1. Cheraskin, E. and Ringsdorf, W. M., Jr.
   Predictive Medicine: A Study in Strategy...A Plan for Maintaining Health by Avoiding Disease
   1973. Mountain View, Pacific Press (hardback)
   1977. New Canaan, Keats Publishing, Inc. (paperback)

   Chapter 10 is designed to emphasize that physical activity influences every aspect of body function—clinical, physiologic, and biochemical or metabolic. In this section, there are examples given to demonstrate relationships between exercise and clinical symptoms and signs, electrocardiographic patterns, biochemical states, and parallelisms between exercise and variables such as coffee/tea, alcohol, tobacco consumption, and vitamin supplementation. In other words, it's clear from this chapter that every cell, tissue, organ and site of the body is directly or otherwise influenced by physical activity.

2. Cheraskin, E., Ringsdorf, W. M., Jr., Medford, F. H., and Hicks, B. S.
   Physical Activity and Carbohydrate Metabolism
   American Laboratory 7: #8, 70-73, August 1975.

It's noteworthy that very little attention has been directed to the relationship of physical activity and carbohydrate metabolism. The few published studies suggest that physical activity serves as a hypoglycemic (blood lowering) agent in hyperglycemic (high blood glucose) subjects. This report is designed to reexamine carbohydrate metabolism in terms of reported physical activity. An attempt was made to analyze the classical 3-hour glucose tolerance test and the diurnal blood glucose patterns in daily exercisers and nonexercisers. It's abundantly clear that there are fewer fluctuations in blood glucose suggesting greater homeostasis in exercisers versus nonexercisers.

3. Cheraskin, E., Ringsdorf, W. M., Jr., Michael, D. W., and Hicks, B. S.
The Exercise Profile
Journal of the American Geriatrics Society 21: #5, 208-215, 1973.

Dietary intake and physical activity were assessed in approximately 700 members of the health professions. It was found that although the diets of both exercisers and nonexercisers contained about the same number of calories, there was a great difference in the proportions of nutrients. For the exercisers, the intake of every vitamin, mineral and amino acid studied exceeded that for the nonexercisers, and many of the differences were statistically significant. The nonexercisers consumed more refined carbohydrates than did the exercisers; the difference was highly significant statistically.

4. Cooper, K. H.
   Aerobics
   1968. New York, Bantam Books.

   This is the first book published on the subject of aerobics. The simple scientific plan provides you with how much and what exercises are available. Based on a then revolutionary new point system that lets you test yourself, figure out how much activity you need, choose your plan and actually measure your progress.

5. Cooper, K. H. and Cooper, M.
   The New Aerobics for Women
   1988. New York, Bantam Books.

   This book is a comprehensive guide to total fitness and particularly for today's woman. Designed for every age and stage of a female's life, Dr. Cooper's uniquely personalized workout plans will help you find the program that is right for you—and your lifestyle. It's of interest that this book includes the unusual questionnaire earlier cited in this chapter.

6. Farquhar, J. W.
   The American Way of Life Need Not be Hazardous to Your Health
   1978. New York, W. W. Norton & Company.

   The author, who established the Stanford Heart Disease Prevention Program in 1972, devotes this entire book to an analysis of the risk factors associated with the epidemic problem of heart disease. Relevant here in this chapter is a portion of a questionnaire which provides a simple measure of the adequacy of a walking agenda to overall health and sickness.

7. Kuntzleman, C. T.
Rating the Exercises: How to Choose the Exercise that Suites You Best
1987. New York, William Morrow & Company

   The author in conjunction with the Editors of Consumer Guide, have created this unusual book designed to provide the reader with an objective appraisal of the pros and cons of just about all forms of exercise from aerobics to yoga. The virtues of the different programs are reported on a star basis. It's noteworthy that walking is rated a four-star activity and therefore for health purposes comparable to any of the more strenuous and exotic programs.

8. Payne W. A. and Hahn, D. B.
Understanding Your Health
1986. St. Louis, Times Mirror/Mosby College Publishing

   This is a contemporary college textbook for health education. It embraces all of the lifestyle considerations. There are a number of interesting self-administrable and self-scorable questionnaires including an overall physical fitness locus of control form. One four-question test is included in this chapter because it provides a quick and easy relatively accurate measure of physical activity.

9. Pleas, J.
   Walking is...
   1981. Nashville, OSSAT, Inc.

   This book is an alternative to the current exercise hodgepodge sweeping the country. The author outlines with unmatched humor the negatives (you cannot expect a Hollywood contract within the first year, straight A's without studying) and many positives (you'll develop a calm personality and acquire a delightful addiction). Additionally, there's a simple qualitative questionnaire which may provide the reader with some measure of the benefits of a leisurely stroll.

10. Prentice, W. E., and Mucher, C.A.
    Fitness for College and Life, 2nd edition
    1988. St. Louis, Times Mirror/Mosby College Publishing

    The second edition of this book is designed to provide a comprehensive, contemporary text for use in classes that are aimed at acquainting college students and adults in general with the nature and score of fitness and to establish acceptable lifelong patterns. It's particularly relevant here because it includes a sample 13-week walking program for beginners. Finally, the questionnaire utilized in this chapter was cited in this book and adapted from Payne and Hahn.

11. Stewart, G. W.
    Every Body's Fitness Book: A Simple, Safe, and Sane Approach to Personal Fitness
    1980. New York, Doubleday.

    The author uniquely provides without personal prejudice a smorgasbord of activity programs and includes a chapter on the most physiologic form of activity, namely walking. Additionally, this book is unique in that it includes the PAR-Q questionnaire which is outlined for completion by the reader.

12. Stutman, F. A.
    The Doctor's Walking Book: How to Walk Your Way to Fitness and Health
    1980. New York, Ballantine Books.

    The author, a medical physician, views walking as the perfect exercise. As justification, he cites numerous biochemical, clinical and psychologic benefits. Included also is a bibliography of exercise books in general and walking in particular.

13. Yanker, G. D.
    Rockport's Complete Book of Exercise Walking
    1983. Chicago, Contemporary Books.

    The uniqueness of this book is that exercise walking means converting the walking you already do—strolling, hiking, backpacking, stair climbing, brisk walking—into exercise routines while preserving the fun of the activity. This text is for moderates. Walkers are not fanatics like other sports or exercise enthusiasts. Walking itself calms you down and gives you an even-handed view of life and exercise. Walking is both emotional and logical. In this monograph, science and art walk together toward a common goal. The logic of this book is like the logic of exercisewalking; the marriage of health and joy.

18

SLEEP: THE OTHER THIRD OF YOUR LIFE

Why a third?

Two reasons.

Somehow the public has recognized that the desirable, preferred, healthy, ideal (call it what you will) sleep state should be about eight hours. That's obviously the **soft** evidence. The **hard** data comes from the scientific literature. For example, E. S. Hammond reported on mortality and sleep habits at the American Public Health Association meeting in 1962. From a study of over 1,000,000 subjects, he discovered the lowest mortality is found in those sleeping seven hours per night. Death rates progressively increased with fewer and with more sleeping hours. Specifically, the highest mortality figures were observed in those with less than five hours and more than ten hours sleep per day. The important point is that approximately one third of the 24 hour interval seems to be the **ideal** sleep period.

As one might expect, there are all kinds of razzle-dazzle classifications of sleep disorders. Fortunately, for our purposes, we can simplify the problem. On the one hand, there are those who have difficulty falling or staying asleep. We call these individuals **insomniacs**. Secondly, there are those who have trouble staying awake. The highfalutin term is **narcolepsy**. Finally, there are various-named syndromes which have as a common denominator a disturbance in the quality of sleep. The **restless-leg** syndrome is but one example.

Are you suffering with insomnia? Take the following questionnaire which was developed by the Sleep Disorders Center of Alabama at Baptist Medical Center Montclair in Birmingham. We acknowledge permission to reproduce their form (Pamphlet CRA 8-87).

		yes	**no**
1.	Thoughts race through my mind and this prevents me from sleeping.	☐	☐
2.	I wake up during the night and can't go back to sleep.	☐	☐
3.	I worry about things and have trouble relaxing.	☐	☐
4.	I wake up earlier in the morning		

		yes	no
	than I would like to.	☐	☐
5.	I lie awake for half an hour or more before I fall asleep.	☐	☐
6.	I feel sad and depressed; I feel afraid to go to sleep.	☐	☐

If you checked affirmatively all six boxes, the chances are very good that you're suffering with insomnia. Obviously, there are shades of grey for this problem. Fewer positive checks may suggest the subtle ramifications of this particular sleep disorder.

It might be of interest to you to know that the generally available figures suggest that somewhere between 10 and 25% of Americans report this problem. And by the way, the female is twice as likely to be affected. Finally, the insomniac will tell you it takes about one hour to fall asleep. Don't believe it. It actually is only about 15 minutes.

The consensus is that one out of three Americans has some kind of sleep disorder. Many of these people suffer needlessly because they are unaware that they have a problem. An excellent example includes those who have difficulty staying awake. Are you a narcoleptic? Take the following test which also was developed by the Sleep Disorders Center at Montclair.

		yes	no
1.	When I experience strong emotions such as anger, fear, or surprise, I go limp.	☐	☐
2.	I have fallen asleep while driving— even after a full night's sleep.	☐	☐

		yes	no
3.	I experience vivid dream-like scenes upon or soon after falling asleep.	☐	☐
4.	I have fallen asleep during physical effort.	☐	☐
5.	I feel as though I have to cram a full day into every hour to get anything done.	☐	☐
6.	I have trouble at work or school because of sleepiness.	☐	☐
7.	I often feel totally paralyzed (unable to move) for brief periods when falling asleep or just after awakening.	☐	☐

As with insomnia, there are obvious gradations of narcolepsy. The more items you checked positive, the greater the possibility of suffering with this disorder. In any case, you're not alone. It's estimated that there are 500,000 narcoleptics. It may be a familial problem suggesting either genetic or environmental contributors. (The nature/nurture debate has been discussed in Chapters 13 and 14.)

Finally, there are those people with problems that are more qualitative. In other words, they sleep poorly and don't awaken with the usual feeling of restfulness. Several disorders have been described by somnologists. One of the most common is termed the restless-leg syndrome. Check the next questionnaire which was also prepared by the Montclair Sleep Center.

		yes	no
1.	Even though I slept through the night, I still feel sleepy during the day.	☐	☐
2.	Other than when exercising, I still experience muscle tension, aching, or crawling sensations in my legs.	☐	☐
3.	I have been told that I kick at night.	☐	☐
4.	I experience leg pain during the night.	☐	☐
5.	Sometimes I can't keep my legs still at night. I just **have** to move them.	☐	☐
6.	I awaken with sore or aching muscles.	☐	☐

The scoring is the same as earlier described. Six yeses suggest that the problem exists. More likely, there will be fewer affirmative responses indicating the gradations of the problem.

Viewed another way, if you're not an insomniac nor a narcoleptic nor one with the restless leg syndrome and related disorder, then the chances are very good that your sleep habits are adequate.

But if you have a problem, what next?

The one thing for certain is that sleep disorders are more often than not multifactorial...meaning that a number of factors are probably serving as contributors.

There's now ample evidence that there are habits which are disruptive to sleep; others are beneficial. The following questions have been adapted from a sleep hygiene test form developed by P. Lacks and M. Rotert. (Reprinted with permission from Behavioral Treatment for Persistent Insomnia by Patricia Lacks, Ph.D., copyright 1987, Pergamon Press, plc) Check these statements.

		yes	no
1.	I take daytime naps.	☐	☐
2.	I go to bed hungry.	☐	☐
3.	I go to bed thirsty.	☐	☐
4.	I smoke more than one pack of cigarettes a day.	☐	☐
5.	I use sleep medication regularly (prescription or over-the-counter)	☐	☐
6.	I exercise strenuously within 2 hours of my bedtime.	☐	☐
7.	I consume food, beverages, or medications containing caffeine.	☐	☐
8.	I drink 3 ounces of alcohol in the evening (e.g. 3 mixed drinks, 3 beers, 3 glasses of wine).	☐	☐

If you answered yes to all eight questions, it's likely that these are the bases for your poor sleep. The obvious solution is to eliminate them...all or some and then check to see the changes in your sleep state.

In contradistinction to these just-cited negative factors, there are other positive lifestyle characteristics which make for good sleep. These have also been developed by Lacks and Rotert. Check your answers.

		yes	no
1.	I sleep approximately the same length of time each night.	☐	☐
2.	I set aside time to relax before bedtime.	☐	☐
3.	I exercise in the afternoon or early evening.	☐	☐
4.	I wake up at the same time each day.	☐	☐
5.	I go to bed at the same time each day.	☐	☐

But your solutions may not be as simple as has been pictured here. True it may be as obvious as eliminating tobacco and/or alcohol or changing your eating habits. (You may already have checked these out in the appropriate chapters.)

There's one more consideration, you may be a **morning** or an **evening person**. As we all know, some of us, jokingly or otherwise, think of ourselves as **owls** and others as **larks**. Most of us are somewhere in between and usually can easily manipulate our sleep-wake cycle to adjust to weekends, shift work, or jet lag with only a modicum of difficulty. So, try this questionnaire designed by J. A. Horne and O. Ostberg which appeared in the International Journal of Chronobiology in 1976. The questionnaire is a translation and adaptation of a questionnaire developed by Professor Ostberg in Sweden. Although this version was developed for use in U.K., it has proved very useful in several U.S. investigations. We here acknowledge the permission granted us to reproduce this material.

Be sure to answer **all** questions. Try to respond to each question independently of all others. Don't go back and recheck. You'll note for questions 1 through 14, the appropriate score for each response is shown in parenthesis. For example, for question 1, if your answer was fairly dependent, then your score would be 2.

1. If there is a specific time at which you have to get up in the morning, to what extent are you dependent on being woken up by an alarm clock?
   Not at all dependent (4)
   Slightly dependent (3)
   Fairly dependent (2)
   Very dependent (1)

2. Assuming adequate environmental conditions, how easy do you find getting up in the mornings?
   Not at all easy (1)
   Not very easy (2)
   Fairly easy (3)
   Very easy (4)

3. How alert do you feel during the first half hour after having woken in the mornings?
   Not at all alert (1)
   Slightly alert (2)
   Fairly alert (3)
   Very alert (4)

4. How is your appetite during the first half-hour after having woken in the mornings?
   Very poor (1)

Fairly poor (2)
Fairly good (3)
Very good (4)

5. During the first half-hour after having woken in the morning, how tired do you feel?
Very tired (1)
Fairly tired (2)
Fairly refreshed (3)
Very refreshed (4)

6. When you have no commitments the next day, at what time do you go to bed compared to your usual bedtime?
Seldom or never later (4)
Less than one hour later (3)
1-2 hours later (2)
More than two hours later (1)

7. You have decided to engage in some physical exercise. A friend suggests that you do this one hour twice a week and the best time for him is between 7:00-8:00 a.m. Bearing in mind nothing else but your own "feeling best" rhythm how do you think you would perform?
Would be in good form (4)
Would be in reasonable form (3)
Would find it difficult (2)
Would find it very difficult (1)

8. You wish to be at your peak performance for a test which you know is going to be mentally exhausting and lasting for two hours. You are entirely free to plan your day and considering only your own "feeling best" rhythm which **one** of the four testing times would you choose?

8:00-10:00 AM (6)
11:00 AM-1:00 PM (4)
3:00-5:00 PM (2)
7:00-9:00 PM (0)   ☐

9. If you went to bed at 11:00 p.m. at what level of tiredness would you be?
Not at all tired (0)
A little tired (2)
Fairly tired (3)
Very tired (5)   ☐

10. For some reason you have gone to bed several hours later than usual, but there is no need to get up at any particular time the next morning. Which **one** of the following events are you most likely to experience?
Will wake up at usual time and will **not** fall asleep (4)
Will wake up at usual time and will doze thereafter (3)
Will wake up at usual time but will fall asleep again (2)
Will **not** wake up until later than usual (1)   ☐

11. One night you have to remain awake between 4:00-6:00 a.m. in order to carry out a night watch. You have no commitments the next day. Which **one** of the following alternatives will suit you best?
Would **not** go to bed until watch was over (1)
Would take a nap before and sleep after (2)
Would take a good sleep before and nap after (3)
Would take **all** sleep before watch (4)   ☐

12. You have to do two hours of hard physical work.

You are entirely free to plan your day and considering only your own "feeling best" rhythm which **one** of the following times would you choose?
8:00-10:00 AM (4)
11:00 AM-1:00 PM (3)
3:00-5:00 PM (2)
7:00-9:00 PM (1) ☐

13. You have decided to engage in hard physical exercise. A friend suggests that you do this for one hour twice a week and the best time for him is between 10:00-11:00 p.m. Bearing in mind nothing else but your own "feeling best" rhythm how well do you think you would perform?
Would be in good form (1)
Would be in reasonable form (2)
Would find it difficult (3)
Would find it very difficult (4) ☐

14. One hears about "morning" and "evening" types of people. Which **one** of these types do you consider yourself to be?
Definitely a "morning" type (6)
Rather more a "morning" than an "evening" type (4)
Rather more an "evening" than a "morning" type (2)
Definitely an "evening" type (0) ☐

For items 15 through 18, make a cross on the scale for your answer. The appropriate score is below the scale. For example, in question 15, if you prefer arising at 7:00 a.m., then place a 4 in the appropriate box.

15. Considering only your own "feeling best" rhythm,

at what time would you get up if you were entirely free to plan your day?

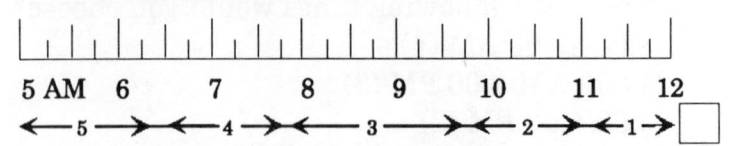

5 AM   6   7   8   9   10   11   12

←―5―→ ←―4―→ ←―― 3 ――→ ←―2―→ ←1→ ☐

16. Considering only your own "feeling best" rhythm, at what time would you go to bed if you were entirely free to plan your evening?

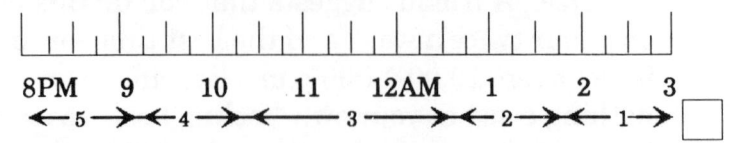

8PM   9   10   11   12AM   1   2   3

←―5―→ ←―4―→ ←―― 3 ――→ ←―2―→ ←―1―→ ☐

17. At what time in the evening do you feel tired and as a result in need of sleep?

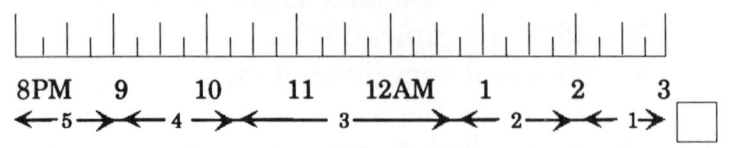

8PM   9   10   11   12AM   1   2   3

←―5―→ ←―4―→ ←―― 3 ――→ ←―2―→ ←― 1―→ ☐

18. At what time of the day do you think that you reach your "feeling best" peak?

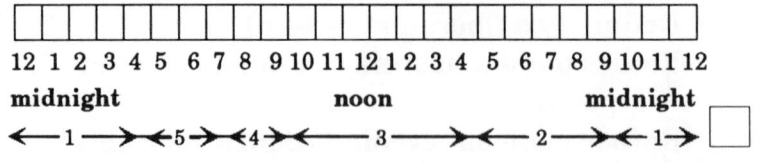

12 1 2 3 4 5 6 7 8 9 10 11 12 1 2 3 4 5 6 7 8 9 10 11 12
midnight   **noon**   **midnight**

←―1―→ ←5→ ←4→ ←―― 3 ――→ ←―― 2 ―→ ←―1―→ ☐

For this last question #19, use the last cross you made (the one on the extreme right hand side) as the reference point. The appropriate score below that point is the one to use. For example, if you select the five consecutive hours to be 9:00 a.m. to 2:00 p.m., then your score would be 2.

19. Suppose that you can choose your own work hours. Assume that you worked a **five**-hour day (including breaks) and that your job was inter-

esting and paid by results. Which **five consecutive hours** would you select?

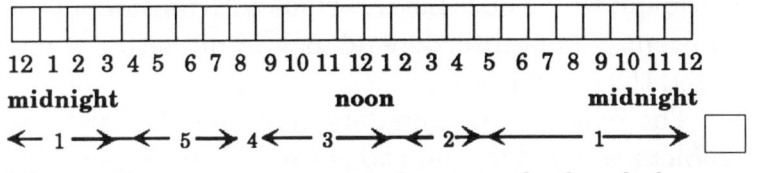

```
┌─────────────────────────────────────┐
└─────────────────────────────────────┘
12 1 2 3 4 5  6 7 8  9 10 11 12 1 2 3 4  5  6 7 8  9 10 11 12
midnight              noon                  midnight
```
← 1 → ← 5 → ← 4 ← 3 → ← 2 → ←—— 1 ——→ ☐

Now add up your scores and put in the box below:

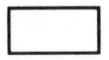

☐

Are you an owl or lark?

A grade of 70 to 86 means you are definitely a morning type. You probably find that your performance peaks in the early hours and rapidly falls as evening approaches. You may have extreme difficulty in adjusting to shift work, jet lag, and changing schedules.

If you're like most people, you probably scored in the 59 to 69 range which is moderately morning type or the 42 to 58 spread which is neither or even 31 to 41 which is the moderately evening subset. This means you can probably manipulate your sleep-wake cycle to adjust to weekends, shift work and to jet lag with only a moderate degree of difficulty.

However, with a score of 16 to 30, you're definitely an evening person. Your body is set for peak functioning at night. Adjustment to shift-work and to jet-lag is probably easier for you than for most people.

In a more practical vein, both extremes **owls and larks** may find it difficult to stay in synch with the other members of your families or with work schedules. The good news is that whether you are an owl or lark it is possible to reset your clock so that you fall into the normal range.

From the extensive and countless cross-references, it should be evident that there's scarcely a problem which does not interface with other problems; a solution not connected with another solution; a problem which does not interface with most if not all solutions. This interdependency is no better illustrated than right here.

The evidence is complete that there's hardly a problem which does not interfere with sleep (e.g. the insomnia associated with rheumatism). There's scarcely a lifestyle characteristic that stands alone. On the one hand, sleep may indeed be a problem; at the very time it can well serve as a solution.

You would be well served to examine the resources carefully. They will provide invaluable information.

RESOURCES

1. American Medical Association
   Guide to Better Sleep
   1984. New York, Random House

    The aim of this text is to summarize the latest scientific research in the field of somnology. The monograph is divided in three parts dealing in order with normal sleep, troubled sleep and better sleep. The chapters are laced with critical philosophic and practical points.

2. Goldberg, P. and Kaufman, D.
   Natural Sleep: How to Get Your Share
   1978. Emmaus, Rodale Press

    This book is a comprehensive guide for people

with sleeping disorders who wish to solve their problem by natural (orthomolecular) means. The authors outline practical solutions. Of particular interest and relevance to this chapter is the extensive discussions of the role of diet/nutrition in sleep mechanisms.

3. Guilleminault, C.
Sleeping and Waking Disorders: Indications and Techniques
1982. Menlo Park, Addison-Wesley Publishing Company

This scholarly work was sponsored by the Association of Sleep Disorders Centers which commissioned the Committee on Somnology and Clinical Polysomnography to assemble under the leadership of C. Guilleminault, M. D. a group of experts for the purpose of putting together the most recent developments in one text. The item of greatest interest in this chapter is the 863 question form developed by Laughton Miles, M. D., Ph. D.

4. Hales, D.
The Complete Book of Sleep: How Your Nights Affect Your Days
1981. Reading, Addison-Wesley Publishing Company

This book, designed for lay educational purposes, translates the latest findings of the new sleep science into a practical and fascinating look at the nights of our lives. Included is a detailed explanation of 42 sleep problems—from snoring and jet lag to breathing problems and insomnia. For the 10 percent of all adults who take sleeping pills each night incorporated is a complete directory of brand-name pills (discussing their effectiveness).

5. Hammond, C. E.
    Some Preliminary Findings on Physical Complaints from a Prospective Study of 1,064,004 Men and Women
    American Journal of Public Health 54: #1, 11-23, January 1964.

    The author, a statistician for the Medical Affairs Department of the American Cancer Society presented this information, from a study of over one million subjects, at the Ninetieth Annual Meeting of the American Public Health Association in 1962. Of particular relevance here are the relationships between number of hours of sleep and mortality. The evidence seems clear that the highest death rate occurs in subjects with the fewest number of hours of sleep (less than five). Also, high mortality figures occurred in those sleeping 10+ hours. The parabolic pattern is further emphasized by the lowest death rate in those with a seven hour sleep pattern per night.

6. Horne, J. A. and Ostberg, O.
    A Self-Assessment Questionnaire to Determine Morningness-Eveningness in Human Circadian Rhythms

International Journal of Chronobiology 4: 97-110, June 1976.

The purpose of this report was to further assess the concept of morningness-eveningness and to design and evaluate an English language morningness-eveningness quiz. This is the background report for the questionnaire cited in this chapter.

7. Lacks, P.
Behavioral Treatment for Persistent Insomnia
1987. Elmsford, Pergamon Press

The author, a practicing psychologist, reviews briefly the physiology and psychology of sleep. For our purposes, the most fascinating section consists of a series of self-administrable and self-scorable sleep hygiene questionnaires. These are intended to provide the reader with an estimate of his or her knowledge of problems contributing to sleep disorders.

8. Mattlin, E.
Sleep Less, Live More
1979. New York, Lippincott

The author attempts to explode the 8-hour a night sleep routine. This is accomplished with a 14-point program for cutting down on sleep while waking up better rested and more energetic. He contends that most of us could sleep at least an hour and a half less each night without adversely affecting our physical and emotional well-being in the slightest and we would save 547 hours a year! Hours you could devote to all those cherished projects you simply can't find the time for.

9. Regestein, Q. R. and Rechs, J. R.
   Sound Sleep
   1980. New York, Simon and Schuster

   There are two important reasons for including this book. On the one hand, it provides a number of self-administering and self-scoring questionnaires which can enlarge the reader's knowledge of his or her own sleeping habits. Additionally, the book is unique in that it provides material to rate the phenomenon of arousability in sleep disorders.

19

OTHER SOLUTIONS

This is the time (in this last chapter of the section) to try to tidy up our thoughts with regard to the place of solutions in **health and happiness**.

Surely the evidence is abundantly clear that a host of lifestyle changes can significantly solve many of our problems. We've devoted already considerable attention to physical activity (Chapter 17), tobacco and alcohol (Chapters 15 and 16), and sleep (Chapter 18).

And we've surely examined diet/nutrition (Chapter 14)!

We hope that by now, the point has been made that **good** diet makes for **good** health; **bad** diet leads to **bad** health. While in general terms this statement stands, it's clearly an oversimplification. What is good and bad diet has changed significantly with industrialization and its consequences upon civilization.

Did you know?
- At the time of George Washington, the average American consumed 2 pounds of sugar per year; today it's climbed to approximately 120 pounds
- We eat a third less fresh fruit than we did in 1936, but three times as much dried, canned, chilled, and frozen fruit
- The typical American takes in about one fourth of an ounce of fiber a day, much less than his forbearers did a century ago

Man no longer steps out in the garden and picks his fruits and vegetables. It must now be collected, transported and stored, processed, purchased, rinsed, defrosted, cooked, allowed to stand, through a series of steps from the garden to the gullet which significantly, and usually unfavorably, influences the food quality.

Believe it or not:
- From the kitchen to the steam table, the average potato loses 95% of its vitamin C value
- We eat 44% more frozen vegetables than in 1960
- Oranges of different species grown in different parts of the country may vary in vitamin C concentration by 400%

Finally, this crazy cultural change has been accompanied by the enormous addition of foreign substances (ordinarily totally unfamiliar to the organism). This includes coloring and flavoring agents, preservatives, insecticides and pesticides, blenders, stabilizers, fillers and scores of other strangely labeled chemical substances. While this phenomenon is often understandable and sometimes even justifiable, it raises serious questions about the role of food in **health and happiness**.

Listen to this:
- In 1976, the average American ate 6.9 pounds of saccharin (mostly as an ingredient in prepared foods)
- We consume 10 times as much food coloring as in 1940
- To improve the texture, cosmetics, and shelf-life of their products, America's food processors add 4.5 pounds of additives per person per year

There's really no need for a questionnaire to ascertain the ingestion of these many foreign and potentially hazardous items. On balance, one can say that, all other things being equal, for the reasons given here and elsewhere, **packaged** foods are less desirable than **natural** products. A simple warning, if you can't pronounce the chemicals on the label, don't eat the food!

There's one more point to be resolved about food. Is it possible to prioritize lifestyle? For example, we know that man can live without food for weeks or even months. In contrast, without water, life ceases in a matter of days.

As a matter of fact, did you know this about body water composition:
- losing only 1% can cause thirst or pain
- a 5% decrease invites hallucinations
- With a drop of 15% there's death!

For these and other reasons, it's obviously time to examine the water we drink (or should we say eat?).

As far as we can determine, there are no known daily water requirements. For one, the state of the art leaves much to be desired. Secondly, the problem is complicated by a number of variables. Water may be consumed in many beverages such as coffee, tea, carbonated drinks, alcohol, etc.

Are you aware that in America:
- Four out of 5 adults drink coffee, and they each average 3 1/3 cups a day
- Each person consumes about a bottle of pop a day—to be precise that's three times as much as he/she drank in 1954
- Would you believe in 1879, the typical American imbibed three bottles of pop a year!

The story is complicated by the fact that it's difficult to estimate the water content of foods.

For example, did you know?
- the water content of cucumbers is 96%
- lettuce is just below that with 95%
- on the other hand, pretzels have only 8% water
- and would you believe, popcorn is a mere 4%

The general consensus is that the average sedentary person needs about 6 to 8 glasses of water on a daily basis. It's obvious that we don't need a questionnaire. You have a good idea of how close you come to the suggested optimal intake. If you're not in this range then water per se may be a problem. Altering your habits and increasing your water intake will clearly be the solution.

Does this solve our water problem? Resoundingly, no! Not only do we need a critical amount; but it must be of good quality. In other words, how safe are our water supplies? What are the connections between water and **health and happiness**?

Did you know?
- 1000 organic contaminants have now been identified in drinking water
- in a study of over 100 municipal water supplies, the evidence is clear that as water hardness goes down, heart disease goes up

There's no argument but that the usual available water supplies leave much to be desired. Hence, there's no question but that our present water supplies constitute a serious problem for **health and happiness**.

What are the solutions? On the one hand, efforts must be made by governmental agencies to do what is necessary (and what is needed in many cases is well established) to provide us with healthful water. On the other hand, there's much that we as individuals can do. For one, we can resort more to bottled water.

Are you aware that?
- sales of bottled water are growing more quickly than those of any other drink
- one out of six households uses bottled water

There are bottled waters and bottled waters ...approximately 300 different bottling plants producing more than 400 diverse brands of water with all kinds of varied claims and counterclaims. What these bottled products have in common is that they purport not to have the terrible contaminants confirmed in our regular water supplies.

Additionally, we can improve our water by changing our dietary habits. We've just learned that some foods are very high in water content; others low. Interestingly, all other things being equal, the healthful foods are in the former category. Specifically, this includes fresh fruits and vegetables.

For more particulars regarding diet and water,

you might want to reexamine your own eating habits (Chapter 14).

Finally, something must be said about air. And this is so because of oxygen (O_2). You'll recall that one can live for months without food and days without water...but with no air death follows in minutes.

But there are other and exciting aspects of air not usually considered. To begin with there's the observation that light, and specifically ultra violet (UV) rays, enters the eye. Through still-to-be-understood mechanisms, it exerts far reaching and generally not recognized reverberations.

Quite apart, since the beginning of time, there's been evidence to suggest that a **healthy** life means getting up with the chickens at the crack of dawn and retiring with them at dusk. Implied if not literally stated is that the **good** life is in some way connected to light. This must be equated against modern man who shuts himself away in an office and scarcely sees the light of day. Does this in any way create **problems** and by changing ones lifestyle (meaning more light) does light become a **solution**?

The answer is a resounding yes!

For example,

- In 1959, 14 out of 15 cancer patients exposed to more sunlight showed unusual evidence of slowing of the malignant process
- Hyperkinetic children provided with more natural light in a classroom demonstrated obvious amelioration of their unusual behavior
- Kids provided with more natural light exhibited 20 to 33% less tooth decay during a one year experimental period

How big a problem (and therefore how much of a solution) comes from an awareness of the importance of natural illumination?

As man has become more industrialized, living under an environment of artificial light, behind window glass and windshield, watching TV, looking through colored sunglasses, working in windowless buildings, the wavelength energy entering the eye has become greatly distorted from that of natural sunlight. Notwithstanding, today the lighting in virtually all research laboratories is still the responsibility of the janitor and is classified as ordinary building maintenance. Those in charge of most research labs seldom acknowledge that light has any biologic effect on laboratory animals or people, and they criticize and ridicule the few scientists who do recognize its importance.

Doctor John Nash Ott, in the opinion of many of us the father of photobiology, provides in two of his books (mentioned in the reference material at the end of this chapter) startling evidence that light may be a critical variable in cancer research and treatment. He also contends that hyperactivity and irritability in some children may be related to the kind of fluorescent lighting used in the classroom. Further, he suggests that full-spectrum sunlight does possess the healthful and healing properties historically ascribed to it, if it's not blocked from entering the eye.

Is this your problem? You don't really need a quiz to find out. All other things being equal, an **indoor** person will probably have a greater light deficit than an **outdoor** type. If you sit at a desk all day, rarely go out to lunch, wear spectacles and especially sun glasses, sit in front of the boob tube all weekend, then you're likely to be suffering with the consequences of inadequate light. The solution? There are all kinds of possibilities. For instance, one can switch jobs to provide more outdoor time. On the other hand, you can substitute full-spectrum glasses (which provide more natural light). Finally, there are more drastic measures, such as replacing the windows in your home with full spectrum material so that it allows the transmission of ultra violet rays.

Problem two. If you're a newsfreak, then you know the nuclear age is upon us. Actually, our society has been in the nuclear business since the atomic bomb was first developed at the end of World War II. It's potential was heightened when it was dropped on the Japanese cities of Hiroshima and Nagasaki. There's no question that there are great benefits. One is that it reduces our dependency on fossil fuels as energy sources. Additionally, nuclear energy can (and already does) improve our industrial and medical technology. This is evidenced by an expanding use of radioactive materials in the diagnosis and treatment of various medical disorders.

But there's a price. The negative health effects that come from day-to-day exposure to radiation. (To understand this let's look at the radiation language.) For our purposes, we'll be dealing with units called rem and millirem (mrem). The rem is a radiation dose unit that measures damaging effect. A millirem is simply 1,000th of a rem. A single dosage of 10,000 mrem (10 rems) or less is generally referred to as low-level radiation; a single dosage of 100,000 mrem (100 rems) or more is considered to be high-level radiation. A dose of 100,000 rems spells sudden death!

Would you like to know what your average annual exposure to radiation is? Fill in the blank spaces in the column on the right in the chart below. (From **Living in the Environment: An Introduction to Environmental Science,** Fourth Edition by G. Tyler Miler, Jr. copyright 1985, 1982 by Wadsworth, Inc. Reprinted by permission of the publisher.)

radiation source	estimated annual dose (in millirems)	
natural radiation:		
Cosmic rays from space At sea level	40.0	(U.S. average)
Add 1 mrem for each 100 feet you live above sea level		(Your risk)
Radiation in rocks and soil (ranges from 30-200)	55.0	(U.S. average)
Radiation from air, water, and food (ranges from 20-400)	25.0	(U.S. average)
Radiation from Human Activities:		
Medical and dental X-rays and treatments	80.0	(U.S. average)
Working or living in a stone or brick building (add 40 for each, if applicable)		(Your risk)
Smoking one pack of cigarettes per day (add 40 mrem)		(Your risk)
Nuclear weapons fallout	4.0	(U.S. average)
Air travel: add 2 mrem a year for each 1500 miles flown		(Your risk)
TV or computer screens—add 4 mrem/year for each 2 hours of exposure per day		(Your risk)
Occupational exposure (depends on job)	0.8	(U.S. average)

Living next to a nuclear power plant (boiling water reactor, add 76 mrem; pressurized water reactor, add 4 mrem ☐ (Your risk)

Living within 5 miles of a nuclear power plant (add 0.6 mrem) ☐ (Your risk)

Normal operation of nuclear power plants, fuel processing, and research facilities $\boxed{0.1}$ (U.S. average)

Miscellaneous—industrial wastes, smoke detectors, certain watch dials $\boxed{2.0}$ (U.S. average)

your total points ☐

How do you compare with others? The average annual exposure per person in the United States is 230 mrem. Of this, 130 mrem generally comes from natural radiation and 100 mrem is derived from human activities. Your exposure may be considerably higher depending on your place of residence, water supply, medical tests and treatments, occupation, and specific health behaviors, including smoking and exposure to sun.

The smallest average exposure to ionizing radiation in the United States comes from nuclear power plants and other nuclear facilities—assuming that they are operating normally. According to the experts, exposure to 1 mrem of ionizing radiation—10 times the average from normally operating nuclear power plants and other nuclear facilities—increases the risk that an individual will die from cancer by about one chance in 8 million. It's been calculated that this risk corresponds to a 1.2 minute reduction in life expectancy and is equivalent to the hazard from taking about 3 puffs on a cigarette (each cigarette reduces life expectancy by about 10 minutes) or an overweight person eating 10 extra calories by taking a small bite from a piece of buttered bread. Similarly, the risk of having a genetically defective child because of exposure to 1 mrem of ionizing radiation received before conception is estimated to be about one chance in 40 million—about 140 times lower than the calculated genetic risk from drinking 29 milliliters (1 fluid ounce) of alcohol and 2.4 times that from consuming one cup of coffee.

One gets the impression from some of these numbers that radiation hazards may be small. However, there's the possibility of a **cumulative** effect. What about, for example, smoking, living next to a nuclear plant, flying frequently, and on and on.

That's the bad news. The good news is that you can **accumulate** a protective lifestyle. For instance, it's possible, as it were, to vaccinate oneself by good eating habits, proper physical activity, reduction in alcohol and tobacco, sensible water intake and healthful sleeping patterns. Obviously, it wouldn't hurt to reduce flying time, changing residence and possibly even switching jobs. As but a small example of one antiradiation solution, the literature recognizes the protective virtues of increased vitamin C supplementation.

And finally, there's still another way of assessing the atmosphere. It (almost) smacks of the occult.

What about this scenario?

The young office worker winced back the pain from a throbbing headache and wondered if the low cloud that had been hovering over midtown Manhattan would disappear by the end of the day. While he massaged his temples, a nonasthmatic waitress (in relatively pollution-free Nebraska) began wheezing and struggling for breath. Meanwhile, half a world away, a Chinese farmer clutched his chest in agony, the victim of a sudden heart attack. Three different people in three different places with nothing in common, except they were all weather-sensitive.

Folklore? Don't bet on it.

Since the days of Hippocrates scientists have been charting physical ailments and mood swings under varying meterologic conditions. And as medicine waltzed into the 20th century, modern researchers began discovering that weather can have a profound physical and psychologic impact on large numbers of people.

Between 1935 and 1972, for instance, more than 70 percent of 120 studies worldwide showed a positive correlation between illness or death and the weather.

Who among us hasn't heard a friend, relative or acquaintance predict a change in weather because "I feel it in my bones," or "my arthritis is acting up again," with startling accuracy? Well, the weather's effect on man and lower animals doesn't stop at the bones. Experts in the field of biometerology (the study of weather and how it relates to health) have pinpointed many physical and emotional states that present themselves under certain conditions in individuals who are weather-sensitive. These circumstances include exhaustion, increased proneness to errors, forgetfulness, visual disturbances, breathing difficulties, depression, insomnia, nervousness, aches in old bone fractures, arthritis pain and even heart attacks.

In one recent issue of the journal Clinical Cardiology, Dr. Tsung O. Cheng, professor of medicine at George Washington University in Washington, D.C., cited the work of a Chinese study that analyzed 943 patients with acute heart attack between 1976 and

1980. The Chinese physicians found a definite increase in heart attacks during the winter months (and this not due to shoveling snow!). They also discovered heart attacks rose under conditions of low humidity.

"That there's a definite meterologic influence on the incidence of acute myocardial infarction (heart attack) seems to be a universal phenomenon. It's very important that such valuable medical information be shared among our cardiologic colleagues around the world," Dr. Cheng concluded.

He isn't alone. In the same journal, Professor G. Ruhenstroth-Bauer, of the world renouned Max-Planck Institutes in West Germany, proclaimed: "the incidence of heart infarcts (attacks) in China confirms a number of older investigations in Europe and shows that these correlations are probably valid around the world." He goes on to point out a 1985 German study that also demonstrated a significant correlation between certain atmospheric conditions and the incidence of heart attack.

While these examples are of a more dramatic nature, it's important to know that anyone who's weather-sensitive could have their **health and happiness** compromised under certain meterologic circumstances.

To give you some idea of how real this problem is, one in every three people are weather sensitive.

Are you one of those who is bound to be under the weather sometimes? The following questionnaire was developed by Volker Faust, M.D., and based on a study of 778 patients in Basel Switzerland between 1972 and 1976. We wish to thank Dr. Faust for granting us permission to reproduce this material.

If you've noticed some relationship between the complaints listed on the quiz and the weather, check the yes column; if not, mark the maybe/no column.

Excluding apparent causes, such as illness, excessive drinking, drug use or other known problems, do you sometimes or often:

		yes	maybe/no
1.	feel tired?	☐	☐
2.	find yourself in a bad mood?	☐	☐
3.	dislike your work more than usual, or dislike all work?	☐	☐
4.	suffer mild headaches?	☐	☐
5.	sleep fitfully?	☐	☐
6.	suffer severe headaches?	☐	☐
7.	find it hard to concentrate?	☐	☐
8.	have trouble falling asleep?	☐	☐
9.	feel unusually nervous?	☐	☐
10.	ache at an old bone fracture?	☐	☐
11.	see flickering spots with eyes open or closed?	☐	☐
12.	notice an increase in forgetfulness?	☐	☐
13.	seem exhausted?	☐	☐
14.	suffer from physical blahs?	☐	☐

	yes	maybe/no
15. wake up, and can't go back to sleep?	☐	☐
16. make many mistakes?	☐	☐
17. suffer spells of dizziness?	☐	☐
18. become aware of rapid or irregular heartbeat?	☐	☐
19. hurt or seriously itch around an old scar?	☐	☐
20. feel depressed?	☐	☐
21. pant or breathe with difficulty?	☐	☐
22. suffer from rheumatic/arthritic pain	☐	☐

You'll remember that some of these questions have earlier cropped up in other quizzes and in connection with other syndromes. However, if you checked the **yes** column for one or more complaints you noticed had a weather connection, an expert like Dr. Faust would probably diagnose you as weather-sensitive.

You'll now notice in the upcoming table the 22 questions have been rearranged in order of decreasing frequency. In other words, tiredness is the number one complaint in weather-sensitive individuals. Specifically, it's noted in 56% of the cases. Conversely, rheumatic/arthritic pains are encountered in 15%. Secondly, you'll find in the column on the extreme right a number which represents how much more often this particular problem is observed in weather-sensitive versus weather-stable individuals. For instance, in the first question, dealing with fatigue, the number 2.7 means that one can expect tiredness 2.7 times more frequently in weather sensitive persons.

rank	symptom	%	factor
1	tiredness	56	2.7
2	bad humor	50	3.4
3	dislike of work	45	2.7
4	mild headache	43	3.3
5	disturbed sleep	42	3.1
6	severe headache (migraine)	38	5.4
7	impaired ability to concentrate	38	4.5
8	difficulty falling asleep	35	3.0
9	nervousness	30	3.3
10	pain in old bone fracture	26	3.1
11	visual disturbances (flickering)	22	3.7
12	increased forgetfulness	24	4.4
13	exhaustion	22	5.4
14	general malaise (physical blahs)	21	4.6
15	difficulty sleeping after waking	23	2.6
16	increased proneness to errors	25	3.3
17	vertigo (dizziness)	22	5.5
18	rapid (or irregular) heartbeat	20	5.0
19	scar-related pain (or itch)	20	3.9
20	depression	18	5.8
21	breathing difficulties	16	5.2
22	rheumatic/arthritic pains	15	4.1

There are many exciting and highly scientific documents dealing with the subject of bioclimatology. For the interested reader, we recommend three texts (pages 367 and 370) listed in the appended bibliography.

Obviously, this is not the end. Other significant habits should be included in this potpourri. In the interest of time and space, let's end this discussion with noise. There are obviously noises and noises. Some are pleasant and healing like the chirping of the birds at the farm in the summer; others can be devastating like the pain of an airhammer.

According to the Environmental Protection Agency (EPA), about 20 to 25 million Americans are exposed to noises of sufficient duration and intensity to cause some permanent loss of hearing. Additionally, 5 million children under age 18 suffer with impaired hearing (mostly from listening to loud music from home stereos, portable jam boxes held close to the ear, and earphones). According to the EPA nearly half of all Americans are regularly exposed to levels of noise in their neighborhoods and jobs that interfere with communication, sleeping, and contribute to annoyance and overall displeasure.

Industrial surveys report that noise exposure results in increased anxiety and emotional distress. Workers habitually surrounded by high intensity noise (usually 110 decibels, abbreviated db, or above) show increased incidence of nervous complaints, nausea, headaches, instability, argumentativeness, sexual impotency, changes in general mood and anxiety.

The problem of noise continues to be studied extensively and especially in occupational medicine. Many relevant books are available. These are cited in the reference section (pages 367 and 368).

The solution is obvious! To the extent possible one should avoid situations associated with unpleasant and unhealthy sounds.

It's now time to close the thought emphasized in this chapter and also to bring to an end the concepts dealt with in this section. There's no question but that there are many real **solutions** to our many real **problems**. This has been repeatedly underlined. What perhaps needs reemphasized is that the lifestyle characteristics which make up our solutions may, in themselves be problems. This has been demonstrated abundantly in these pages.

Clearly, many of our lifestyle features are totally under our control. We don't have to consult anybody to decide to quit smoking or quit boozing. In contrast, some other of our lifestyle habits are only partially under our own will. We can, for instance, control considerably what we eat. On the other hand, what's in our food is in good measure (and unfortunately increasingly) determined by others such as the food industry.

Finally, part of our lifestyle is impossible or, for practical purposes, not feasibly modifiable by ourselves. Some of the areas, like noise, have been dealt with in this last chapter. Even more glaring examples of conditions not manageable by the individual appear regularly in the electronic and print media. Obvious examples are ozone, the greenhouse effect, and acid rain.

Now that we've gotten some sense of our problems (Section B) and our solutions (Section C), where do we go from here? How old are we really? This will be the purpose of the epilogue and the answer to the burning question "are you 70 going on 40...or 40 going on 70?."

RESOURCES

1. Gabler, R.
   Is Your Water Safe to Drink?
   1988. Mount Vernon, Consumers Union

   This comprehensive text released by the

Editors of Consumer Reports provides a panoramic picture of the problems of water. Particular attention, in separate chapters, is paid to health hazards in drinking water, such as microbial, inorganic and organic agents and chlorination. For the sophisticated reader there's available extensive bibliographic documentation.

2. Jones, D. M. and Chapman, A. J.
Noise and Society
1984. Chichester, John Wiley & Sons

This book looks at the problem of noise from a number of points of view and is of special interest to the physiologist, engineer, clinician, psychologist, psychiatrist, and jurist. It's particularly relevant here because of a chapter entitled The Effects of Noise on Health with subdivisions dealing with the mental and physical state, mortality, and medical implications of deafness.

3. Kals, W. S.
Your Health, Your Moods and the Weather
1982. New York, Doubleday and Company, Inc.

This well-written, informative book holds a wealth of information on the weather and health. The author offers an easy-to-read introduction to meteorology which is aimed at alerting the reader to weather conditions most likely to contribute to symptoms. Mr. Kals also provides information to help readers learn how to chart, predict and understand their weather related states. In addition, he shows how to ascertain which city in America has the best climate for any particular individual's problem, and suggests ways to minimize the effects of weather on emotions and health—"and how to live with the ones we can't change." Special mention should be made that this book includes an excellent questionnaire which is cited earlier in this chapter.

4. Loeb, M.
Noise and Human Efficiency
1986. Chichester, John Wiley & Sons

Dr. Michael Loeb, as an international authority on noise and hearing, reflects the breadth of his knowledge and interests in auditory phenomena. The manuscript deals with the entire range of noise-related research, from basic acoustics through problems of temporary or permanent deafness, and the effects of noise on speech perception to the impairments or facilitation found in cognitive performance. The book will serve to instruct those who have the motivation to study its subject matter. It'll also function as a reference work.

5. Miller, G. T., Jr.
Living in the Environment, Fourth edition
1985. Belmont, Wadsworth Publishing Company

This book is intended to serve as a simple introductory course in environmental studies in an accurate, balanced, and interesting way. Additionally, the text uses basic ecologic concepts to highlight environmental problems and to indicate possible ways to deal with them. More directly, the monograph contains a section on radiation and includes an informative quiz which is employed earlier in this chapter.

6. Ott, J. N.
Health and Light
1976. New York, Pocket Book

The cardinal point of this fascinating book is that, in a sense, light may be viewed like food, it can be good or bad and understandably make for health or sickness. This was the first lay text designed to study light both natural and artificial. Specific attention is relegated to subjects as diverse as sunglasses, the role of light in arthritis, its contribution to cancer and the connection of fluorescent lighting and tiredness.

7. Ott, J. N.
Light, Radiation and You: How to Stay Healthy
1982. Old Greenwich, The Devin-Adair Company

This book, a follow up of the author's Health and Light, deals in greater detail with earlier studies and introduces new experiments to emphasize the importance of light in **health and happiness**. Topics include controlled exposure to certain colors which can produce, or reduce, aggressive behavior in both human beings and laboratory animals. Hyperactivity and irritability in some children may be related to the kind of fluorescent lighting used in the classroom.

8. Rosen S.
   Weathering: How the atmosphere conditions your body, your mind, your moods—and your health
   1979. New York, M. Evans and Company, Inc.

   This book is a unique accounting of the fascinating subject of weathering. The author provides the latest research as well as historical data. There are examinations of physique, temperament, social class, age and sex and how these factors influence your own weather-sensitivity risk profile. Included is an excellent self-scoring questionnaire.

9. Rosen, S.
   Deep Weather
   Editors of Rodale Press
   Listen to Your Body
   1982. Emmaus, Rodale Press. pp. 20-25

   Dr. Rosen, a scientist who has spent years researching biometeorology, provides a quick glance at weather and health, and offers easy-to-read charts which relate weather to **health and happiness**. Other maps reveal how weather may affect your moods and behavior. There's an excellent questionnaire cited in this book.

THE EPILOGUE

When I embarked on this project the concept of **health and happiness** was no stranger. For about half a century the complexities of that marvelous machine called the human body have been all consuming. The mysteries and magic of wellness served as a focal point.

For the past nineteen chapters, we've been inquiring about your body. We should, by now, know what works and doesn't, how well and, to a degree, why. What we've done is really no different than what you have or will do when you go out to buy a house.

Certainly you'd check the integrity of the foundation, try the heating and air conditioning units and have a look through the attic and basement. Maybe you'd inch your way across the roof, inspecting the drains and then tiles, eventually working your way down to the gutters. You'd certainly check the plumbing for leaks. The soundness of beams and supports would be important too, for without a strong backbone the walls would surely come tumbling down. You would, of course, need to know what to look for, lest the new cosmetic paint job fool you into thinking you're getting something you haven't bargained for. After all, the smart buyer always arms himself with the best available information to get the most return on an investment.

Through **Health and Happiness** you've been offered a simple buyer's guide to provide you the most basic of tools to achieve this end.

By means of the 50 or so quizes you've just completed, you've shown a willingness to identify the multitude of glitches in life's long road. You've obviously completed the first step.

It was not my intent to offer magic bullets, because there are none. **Health and happiness** is there, and it's free, and it's yours...all you have to do is go for it.

And you can go for it by reading the next and last chapter!

20

ARE YOU 40 GOING ON 70 ... OR 70 GOING ON 40?

When I. M. Well (obviously not his real name) stepped through the doorway of a Holiday Inn banquet room his former classmates stared in awe.

Some, swilling down martinis in between puffs on a cigarette while desperately trying to hide the middle-age spread, couldn't believe their eyes.

His skin was taut and glowed a healthy bronze. The bags that drooped beneath the eyes of many in the room were conspicuously absent. His teeth sparkled under the chandeliered lighting.

While some would like to have believed the

skilled hands of a plastic surgeon had turned back the clock for him, the truth is he did it all himself.

"There's nothing mysterious about how I look and feel," he told a former flame who wanted to know his secret. "For starters, I married a wonderful woman, quit smoking years ago, and only drink in moderation. I decided shortly after graduation that I wanted to live life to the fullest and for the longest amount of time that this machine we call the body lasts."

"In other words," he declared, "I want to be 70 going on 40, not 40 going on 70!"

Scenarios like this take place thousands of times in hundreds of cities each day, and those who get the pat on the back all have one thing in common: They look better, feel better and have an enviable gusto because their bodies are younger than their years. Most didn't start turning back the clock right after high school either. The journey generally began in their 30s, 40s, 50s and later.

The scientific and lay literatures gush with a mind-boggling array of startling statistics and critical charts to help plot how long the average American will live and predict how he or she will die.

The most up-to-date studies show the male in America today can expect to live 72 years; the woman should make it to 78 years. These life expectancy ratings put the United States close to 20th for men and about tenth in the world for women. Let's face it, for the richest country in the world (the only one with a TV set for each eye), the one with the so-called best health care delivery system, that's a long way from the top. Iceland and Japan do much better. For example, the Icelandic male lives 74 years; the female 79. Gambia, in East Africa, is at the bottom with 32 years for males and 35 for the woman.

Next, and also importantly, how do Americans die? The answer suggests a lot of the population is committing unintentional (and if you want to be honest, in many cases intentional) suicide. More than 700,000 people in the United States succumb to heart disease each year. In the vast majority, cigarette smoking, poor dietary habits, and sedentary lifestyles will contribute significantly to their ultimate demise. (You may want to check your own habits in earlier chapters.) These same vices will also kill 328,000 cancer patients and 209,000 stroke victims. Motor vehicle accidents are next in line, claiming 55,000. Follow that with diabetes at 39,000, 25,000 suicides, 19,000 homicides, 7,400 each for drowning and fire victims. The list goes on and on.

Thanks to yearly statistical analyses performed by the Federal Bureau of Investigation (FBI), we know where violent crime (which affects health) most likely occurs. If you don't want to be murdered, raped, robbed or sustain aggravated assault, stay away from Newark, Miami, Detroit, Atlanta, Boston, Baltimore, Washington, D.C., Oakland and New York.

Science is even sophisticated enough now to advise you on **how much** you can shorten your life. At the head of the list is being an unmarried male. The best information available suggests this may cut your life short by 3,500 days. The man who smokes, whether he's married or not, will lose 2,250 days. Being 30 percent overweight accounts for 1,300 days, and you can lop off 900 days of living if you are 20 percent overweight. To top it all off, being poor whittles away 700 days.

The bottom line to these dreadful numbers is they tell us about the **quantity** of life, but they also provide good guidelines on how to improve the **quality** of life.

Our hero had the answer to that one long before he reached the class reunion. He knew where he stood healthwise from the beginning and was able to make lifestyle and diet adjustments to keep his biologic machinery running at optimal performance while looking years younger than his chronologic age.

Most of us really don't know how old our body is... if we did, then we might do something about it. The information is out there to help anyone with the desire to start turning back the clock.

So the question on the docket now is: How many calendar years are you and how does that compare with your biologic age? Are you 40 going on 70...or 70 going on 40?

The immediate issue then is to ascertain how many of us are indeed biologically younger and how many are older than our chronologic years. Nedra Belloc, Lester Breslow and Joseph Hochstim distributed a 23 page health inventory to more than 7,000 people living in Alameda County, California and received 6,928 completed questionnaires (86% of the original sample). On the basis of these data, they identified seven principal levels of health and the percentage of respondents in each category. By examining the following summary, you will learn how many people are basically younger and how many are older than their years. Additionally, you can get some idea of where you fit! We want to acknowledge the permission granted to us by these authors for their original contribution and to thank also Harold H. Bloomfield, M.D. and Robert Kory for their adaptation of this material.

level I: severely disabled (7 percent of population).
- do you have trouble feeding yourself?
- dressing yourself?

- climbing stairs?
- getting outdoors?
- have you been unable to work for six months or more?
- did you report any of the above? if yes, you are in this category. if no, continue.

level II: mildly disabled (8 percent of population).
- have you cut down on your hours of work due to illness or disability?
- have you changed your work due to illness or disability?
- have you had to cut down on nonwork activities for six months or longer?
- did you report any of the above? if yes, you are in this category. if no, continue.

level III: chronically ill—severe (9 percent of population).
- has your doctor told you at any time in the past year that you have any of the following?
    - arthritis (rheumatism)
    - asthma
    - cancer
    - chronic bronchitis
    - chronic gall bladder trouble
    - chronic kidney disease
    - chronic liver trouble
    - diabetes
    - duodenal ulcer
    - emphysema
    - epilepsy
    - heart trouble
    - high blood pressure
    - stomach ulcer
    - stroke
    - tuberculosis

- —ulcerative colitis
- do you have a missing hand, arm, foot, leg?
- do you have trouble seeing even with glasses?
- do you have trouble hearing even with a hearing aid?
- did you report any **two** of the above? if yes, you are in this category. if no, continue.

level IV: chronically ill—moderate (19 percent of population).

- do you have any **one** of the conditions listed under Level III? if yes, you are in this category. if no, continue.

level V: symptomatic but not diagnosed (28 per cent of population).

- have you ever experienced any of the following during the last twelve months?
  - —frequent coughing or wheezing
  - —frequent cramps in legs
  - —frequent headaches
  - —heavy chest colds (more than two per year)
  - —pain in back or spine
  - —pain in heart or chest
  - —paralysis or poor coordination of any kind
  - —repeated pain in stomach or rectum
  - —stiffness, swelling, or aching in any joint or muscle
  - —swollen ankles
  - —tightness or heaviness in chest
  - —tire easily, often low in energy
  - —trouble breathing, shortness of breath
  - —chronic sadness or depression, major sleep difficulty

—frequent anxiety or worry
—sexual problems
—major difficulties at work, school, or home
- did you report any of the above? if yes, you are in this category. if no, continue.

level VI: without complaints, but low to moderate energy level (23 percent of population).
- do you have about the same or perhaps less energy than people your age?
- do you sometimes or frequently have trouble falling asleep or staying asleep through the night?
- when you have only four or five hours' sleep, are you worn out the next day?
- are you sometimes or often worn out at the end of the day?
- did you answer yes to any **two** of the above? if yes, you are in this category. if no, continue.

level VII: without complaints, high energy, robust health (6 percent of population).
- would you say that you have more energy than others your age?
- do you only rarely have trouble falling asleep or sleeping throughout the night?
- when you get only four or five hours' sleep, do you feel only somewhat tired the next day?
- do you only rarely feel completely worn out at the end of the day?
- if you answer yes to **three** of the above four questions, you are in this group.

Phrased another way, Level I above describes the 40-going-on-70 individual. Level VII depicts the 70-going-on-40 person. Now, where do you fit?

The questionnaire you're about to fill out is one of many that are available. It's simple, reasonably accurate (though we do have our differences with it) and can provide some exciting conclusions. It was adapted by the staff of **Prevention**, who used as their guide the book **Nutraerobics: The Complete Individualized Nutrition and Fitness Program for Life After 30**, by Jeffrey Bland, Ph.D. We wish to thank Doctor Bland for granting us permission to reproduce this material.

Answer the following 21 questions with a simple yes or no.

		yes	no
1.	blood pressure less than 130/75	☐	☐
2.	cholesterol less than 180	☐	☐
3.	in good physical shape	☐	☐
4.	no history of chronic illness	☐	☐
5.	no breathing problems or asthma	☐	☐
6.	resting pulse rate less than 60 beats/minute	☐	☐
7.	no vision problem	☐	☐
8.	blood pressure greater than 140/90	☐	☐
9.	overweight	☐	☐
10.	cholesterol level greater than 250	☐	☐
11.	smoke more than half pack per day	☐	☐

		yes	no
12.	more than 2 drinks per day	☐	☐
13.	poor recovery after exercise	☐	☐
14.	anemic	☐	☐
15.	reduced immunity	☐	☐
16.	constipated	☐	☐
17.	easily winded or fatigued	☐	☐
18.	resting pulse rate greater than 80 beats/minute	☐	☐
19.	poor short-term memory for age	☐	☐
20.	difficulty with close vision	☐	☐
21.	sexual dysfunction	☐	☐

Now turn back to the first question which deals with whether your blood pressure is less than 130/75. If your answer is less, then insert a -2 in the appropriate box below. The second question relates to your blood cholesterol, if it's less than 180 mark a -1 in the space provided. Continue this format.

yes to first question (-2)	☐
yes to second question (-1)	☐
yes to third question (-1)	☐
yes to fourth question (-2)	☐

yes to fifth question (-1) ☐

yes to sixth question (-1) ☐

yes to seventh question (-1) ☐

total **A** ☐

Questions 1 through 7 are structured in such a way that if you answer yes you should subtract the number of years (shown in parentheses) from your chronologic age. The overall possible subtractions yield 9 years. Let's say you answer yes for all 7, then your biological age at this point is 9 years less than your actual years. Hence, if you answered yes to the first seven questions and you're actually 45 calendar years old it means you're 45 going on 36.

Beginning with 8 and continuing through the 21st question, you're to **add** below the number of years shown if the answer is yes.

yes to question 8 (+2) ☐

yes to question 9 (+3) ☐

yes to question 10 (+1) ☐

yes to question 11 (+2) ☐

yes to question 12 (+1/2) ☐

yes to question 13 (+1) ☐

yes to question 14 (+1/2) ☐

yes to question 15 (+1) ☐

yes to question 16 (+1) ☐

yes to question 17 (+1) ☐

yes to question 18 (+1/2) ☐

yes to question 19 (+1) ☐

yes to question 20 (+1/2) ☐

yes to question 21 (+1/2) ☐

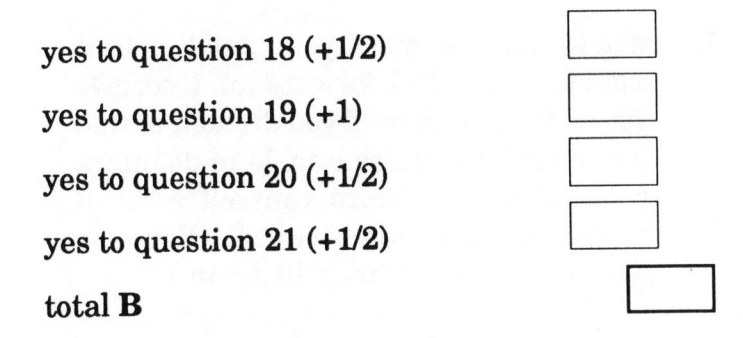

total **B** ☐

The greatest number of years that you can possibly add in this section is 15 1/2. If you answered yes to questions 8 through 21 and are chronologically 45 then adding 15 1/2 makes you 45 going on 60 1/2.

Now enter the scores for sections **A** and **B** of the questionnaire along with your chronologic age to get the grand total for your biological age.

☐ - ☐ + ☐ = ☐
your chronologic age   A   B   your biologic age

Using this simple technique you can derive some notion of whether you are 40 going on 70, 70 going on 40, or any other combination of biologic versus chronologic age.

What does it take to be younger instead of older than your calendar years? You know from reading this book thus far the answer. It lies in analyzing your lifestyle and modifying it by adding well-known and established favorable changes and, at the same time, eliminating undesirable habits and practices.

The following questionnaire (and we wish to thank Dr. Bland for allowing us permission to use this form also) will help you identify the pluses and minuses in your lifestyle.

1. **work**—does it meet your needs? Is it something you look forward to? If so, give yourself a 1.0. Should you dread it or find it's something you're unable to do, mark yourself a 0.0. Score yourself a 0.5 if you're somewhere in between. (You may wish to look at Chapter 10 again.) ☐

2. **recreation and hobbies**—if you know how to relax, enjoy your leisure time, and have adequate recreation and hobbies, give yourself a 1.0. Should you hate vacations, don't know how to occupy your leisure time, and have no recreation, grade yourself a 0.0. Mark down a 0.5 if you're in between. (Why not review Chapter 13?) ☐

3. **pain or suffering**—if you are free from pain or suffering, give yourself a 1.0. Anyone significantly debilitated by pain or suffering, assign yourself a 0.0. In between, 0.5. (It might be wise to reread the early part of this chapter.) ☐

4. **mental suffering, worry, or unhappiness**—if you are free from these, give yourself a 1.0. In the case of considerable unhappiness, worry, tension, and grief, a grade of 0.0 is appropriate. For an in-between situation, mark a 0.5. (Check chapters 8 and 12.) ☐

5. **communication**—if you are able to communicate orally, in writing, and non-verbally to your satisfaction with other people, give yourself a 1.0. Supposing you feel frustrated by lack of communication, people don't listen to you and you can't get things off your chest, allot yourself a 0.0. In the event you're in between, 0.5 would be your grade. (You may wish to consider reviewing Chapter 13.)

6. **sleep**—are you able to get six to eight hours of regular, uninterrupted sleep each night? If so, give yourself a 1.0. With spotty sleep interrupted by insomnia, score yourself a 0.0 accessing a 0.5 for something in between. (If sleep is a problem for you, chapter 18 may provide a solution.)

7. **dependency on others**—if you are usually able to make your own decisions and are operating independently in the world, give yourself a 1.0. In the presence of dependency upon other people and an inability to make decisions for yourself, score a 0.0. Allocate a 0.5 for anything in between. (A review of Chapter 13 might be helpful.)

8. **nutrition**—do you eat a good diet from the seven fundamental food groups each day and maintain an adequate weight-to-

height ratio? If so, give yourself a 1.0. Is your diet more convenience-oriented, high in sugar and fats? Assign yourself a 0.0. Somewhere in between would rate you a 0.5. (For more information on nutrition, see chapter 14.)

9. **excretion**—do you have regular bowel and bladder habits and no problem with constipation? An affirmative answer would afford you a 1.0. However, if you are chronically constipated and need laxatives or have a urinary problem, give yourself a 0.0. On condition that you are in between mark yourself 0.5. (Recheck the early part of this chapter.)

10. **sexual activity**—does your sexual life meet your needs, so that there are no apparent psychological problems? If so, give yourself a 1.0. But if you have apparent sexual problems and/or inadequacy, give yourself a 0.0. With occasional problems, place a 0.5 in the box. (Why not scan Chapter 13 one more time?)

total

After totalling the answers you should have a number ranging between 1 and 10. What does this number mean? The results from this same questionnaire have been studied in over 180 patients and the following relationships between the scores of these patients and their health were found.

If your score was 10 to 8.5, the survey demonstrates relatively good health with a maximum of benign problems.

With grades of 8.5 to 6.5, the evidence suggests the early stages of chronic degenerative diseases.

Marks ranging between 6.5 to 4.0, correlate with gout, diabetes, low back pain and alcoholism.

Finally, in the case of 4.0 to 2.5, the survey reveals acute disease syndromes such as heart failure, cancer, and kidney stones.

Phrased another way and more simply, the higher numbers suggest a favorable discrepancy, namely 70 going on 40; the lower scores above characterized the unfavorable, the 40 going on 70!

For more information, check the following resource section.

RESOURCES

1. Belloc, N. B., Breslow, L. and Hochstim, J. R.
   Measurement of Physical Health in a General Population Study
   American Journal of Epidemiology 93: #4, 328-336, 1971.

   The report, cited in this chapter, presents a refreshing approach to the measurement of health/disease of Alameda County, California, in 1965. Respondents were asked a number of questions regarding disability, chronic conditions, symptoms and energy level. From their responses, they've been categorized along a physical health/sickness spectrum ranging from a minimum state defined by inability to work and/or care for personal needs, to an optimal condition expressed by no complaints and a high level of energy.

2. Bland, J.
    Nutraerobics
    1983. New York, Harper and Row

    Questionnaires that provide an opportunity to learn how to analyze one's own needs and design a personalized lifestyle. The information stems from hundreds of published clinical studies reported by researchers over the years, and clinical experiences with the program in several medical facilities. It's clear that life may not necessarily be prolonged by the information in this book; however, the quality of life as measured by improved health may well be increased.

3. Bloomfield, H. H. and Kory, R. B.
    The Holistic Way to Health and Happiness: A New Approach to Complete Lifetime Wellness
    1978. New York, Simon and Schuster.

    The authors provide an overview of the ingredients for robust health with particular consideration to the personal responsibility factor and nature's healing contributions. Considerable attention is directed to the needed lifestyle alterations. Particular emphasis is placed upon psychosocial aspects (e.g. transcendental meditation).

4. **Blue Cross and Blue Shield Guide to Staying Well**
1982. Chicago, Contemporary Books, Inc.

The book outlines the concerns of this organization regarding the health and sickness of a large segment of the American public. It presents the essentials of lasting good health, nutrition, exercise, other lifestyle characteristics including stress management. It's particularly relevant here for several reasons including the fact that it makes available a self-scoring and grading lifestyle questionnaire.

5. Cheraskin, E. and Ringsdorf, W. M., Jr.
Proneness Profiles in Predictive Medicine
Lab News 4: #1, 24-30, July 1972.

Attempts to predict disease susceptibility have led to the development of proneness profiles. The diagnostic factors include age, sex, weight, blood pressure, blood biochemical values, and dietary habits. Persons with one chronic disorder sooner or later have other chronic ailments. Thus there must be common denominators in seemingly different patterns of proneness. This is illustrated by the well-established coronary proneness profile and by the less well-developed cancer profile. What is urgently needed is a proneness profile designed to anticipate the syndrome of sickness. Such proneness profiles are discussed.

6. Cline, D. W. and Chosey, J. J.
   A Prospective Study of Life Changes and Subsequent Health Changes
   Archives of General Psychiatry 27: #1, 51-53, July 1972.

   The relationship of life events requiring social readjustment to subsequent health change has been examined through the use of the Schedule of Recent Experience in a prospective study of 134 cadets enrolled in an officer training program. Significant positive correlations were found between life and health changes reported on a daily basis for the first two weeks of the training program and for succeeding four- and eight-month periods. The data support the hypothesis that disturbances in social equilibrium parallel changes in physiologic balance.

7. Diamond, H. and Diamond, M.
   Fit for Life. II: Living Health: The Complete Health Program!
   1987. New York, Warner Books.

   This is a highly popular book designed especially for lay-educational purposes. It's a modernized and up-to-date compendium of the commonsense approach of the natural hygiene movement. It addresses in simple language the lifestyle aspects of civilization's killing and crippling problems.

8. Paffenbarger, R. S., and Wing, A. L.

Chronic Disease in Former College Students: XI. Early Precursors of Nonfatal Stroke.
American Journal of Epidemiology 94: #6, 524-530, June 1971.

Doctor-diagnosed stroke was reported by 102 of 10,327 men who had attended Harvard University between 1916 and 1940 and who had returned a usable, self-administered male questionnaire in 1966. Examination of university medical records of these former students revealed four characteristics in youth that predisposed them to increased incidence of nonfatal stroke in later life. They included higher levels of blood pressure, increased weight for height, shorter body stature, and cigarette smoking. Paired combinations of any of the four characteristics demonstrated an additive or greater effect on stroke incidence. High blood pressure exerted the strongest influence on prevalence of nonfatal stroke, both singly and when paired with the three other characteristics.

9. Palmore, E.
Health Practices and Illness Among the Aged
Gerontologist 10: #4, 313-316, Winter 1970.

There's widespread agreement that inactivity, obesity, and cigarette smoking are usually associated with a higher incidence of various illnesses and higher mortality rates. There's corresponding evidence that exercise, weight control, and avoiding cigarettes contribute to the lower incidence of several illnesses and lower death rates. Recently the question has been raised as to whether these health practices are associated with low enough rates of illness among the aged to justify reduced health insurance premiums for those who exercise, display moderate weights and avoid smoking. This paper from the Duke Longitudinal Study of Aging confirms the existence of such an association between health practices and lower rates of illness and death.

10. Pratt, L.
The Relationship of Socioeconomic Status to Health
American Journal of Public Health 61: #2, 281-291, February 1971.

Numerous studies have documented that both the level of health and the quality of personal health behavior are positively related to socioeconomic status. This report primarily tries to answer why the underclass have poorer health than more affluent groups. The data stemming from this experiment tends to support the general proposition that one of the mechanisms through which poverty adversely affects health is a more deficient pattern of personal health care among the poor. This research also found that when low-income women had sound health practices, their health level was as good as that found among high-income females with the same health habits.

11. Stokes, B.
    Self-Care: A Nation's Best Health Insurance
    Science 205: #4406, 547, 10 August 1979.

    At the time this editorial appeared, approximately five million people in the United States belonged to physical or mental self-help groups of some kind—including everything from Alcoholics Anonymous to feminist health collectives. Organized self-care programs have proved especially effective among those suffering chronic illnesses, which represent a growing proportion of the diseases affecting Americans. For example, a diabetics' self-care program sponsored by the University of Southern California reduced the number of patients experiencing diabetic coma by two-thirds and halved the number of emergency room visits. To insure that such a comprehensive health care plan does not lead to even higher medical costs, national insurance should be tied to a program that would encourage people to take more responsibility for their own health. In other words, self-care incentives should be built into all national health plans.

12. Stone I.
    The Healing Factor: Vitamin C Against Disease
    1972. New York, Grossett & Dunlap

    An impressive and formidable account of vitamin C's power to fight illness and disease, including cancer, heart disease, strokes, mental illness, old age, diabetes, arthritis, kidney disease and hepatitis. The author, a noted biochemist, reveals that an ancient genetic mutation has left man without the ability to produce ascorbic acid. Massive documentation shows how this book may ultimately result in better health for human beings. Written in laymen's language, it's an invaluable resource.

13. Wiley, J. A. and Camacho, T. C.
Life-Style and Future Health Evidence from the Alameda County Study.
Preventive Medicine 9: #1, 1-21, January 1980.

A principal aim of research at the Human Population Laboratory (HPL) over the past 25 years has been to investigate the relationship between lifestyle and physical health in the general population. Lifestyle, in this context, consists of discretionary activities which are a regular part of an individual's daily pattern of living. The basic hypothesis underlying this work is that certain components of lifestyle, individually and in combination, exert a significant impact on a person's overall health status. In this report from HPL, it was discovered that certain aspects of daily life were predictive of future health status among survivors in a 9-year longitudinal study. Cigarette smoking, alcohol consumption, physical activity, hours of sleep per night, and weight in relation to height were significantly associated with overall health outcomes 9 years later.

THE INDEX

A

Abrahamson, E. M., 119
Abramson, M., 218
Action on Smoking and Health, 174, 283
Adamson, G. J., 178
Adrenocortical activity, 36
Age
   biologic, 376
   chronologic, 376
Air, 224, 225, 354
Alabaster, O., 47

Alcohol (see Alcoholism)
Alcoholism, 29, 44, 293-311
   CAGE, 295
   MAST, 296-299
   questionnaires, 295, 296-299, 302-303
   rats, 301
   teenagers, 302-303
Alpha Test, 257
American Association of Fitness Directors in Business and Industry, 28
American Bankers Association, 153, 165
American Cancer Society, 42, 174, 274, 283
American Heart Association, 175
American Institute of Cancer Research, 43, 48
American Institute of stress, 176
American Medical Association, 110, 129, 344
American Psychiatric Association's Diagnostic and Statistical Manual (DSM III), 74
Anatomy of an Illness, 4
Anderson, A. E., 82
Anemia, 20
   iron deficiency, 30
Angers Happiness Questionnaire, 219
Anorexia nervosa, 73-78
   EAT, 85-86
   handbook for counselors and therapists, 87
   questionnaire, 78-79
   subclinical, 83
   treatment of, 82, 88
Anorexia Nervosa and Related Eating Disorders, Incorporated (ANRED), 81
Arthritis, 57-71, 369
   aspirin, 66
   diet, 66, 67
   nicotinic acid, 68
   questionnaires, 59-63

tocopherol, 69
Arthritis Foundation (AF), 63
Arthritis Information Service/University of Alabama at Birmingham, 64
Association for Fitness in Business (AFB), 175
Atkinson, H., 30

B

Barnes, B. O., 120
Basta, S. S., 30
Bauer, W., 66
Beck, A. T., 202
Beck Depression Inventory (BDI), 189, 202
Belloc, Nedra, 376, 387
Berkley, G., 66
Bertera, R. L., 240
Bioclimatology, 359, 364
Biometerology, 360
Bjurstrom, L. A., 179
Blair, S. N., 178
Bland, Jeffrey, 380, 388
Blood glucose, 52, 53
Bloomfield, Harold H., 376, 388
Boredom, 24
   fatigue, 37
Bradburn, N. N., 219
Breslow, Lester, 376
Brody, J., 262
Bruch, H., 83
Bruns, C., 143
Bulimia, 73-88
   questionnaire, 78-79
Bumpus, John F., 113
Burkett, Larry, 164
Burn-out, 24

questionnaires, 26, 27, 33, 37, 39
job stress, 36, 38
Bushed, 19
Butterworth, C. E., Jr., 48
Button, E. J., 83

C

CAGE questionnaire, 294-295, 305-306
Cancer, 41-56, 355, 369
    blood glucose, 52
    carbohydrate metabolism, 50, 51
    diet, 53, 54
    folic acid, 48
    how to overcome, 55
    nutrition, 55
    ponderal index, 53
    prevention of, 47
    questionnaires, 43, 48, 54
    vitamin C, 49, 54
    weight, 52
Candidiasis (see yeast infection)
Cameron, E., 49
Carbohydrate metabolism, 50, 51
Carcinoma (see cancer)
Carpenter, Karen, 75
Center for Corporate Health Promotion, Inc., 177
Center for Health Promotion and Education, 29
Center for Science in the Public Interest, 249
Center for the Study of Anorexia and Bulimia, 81
Center of Alcohol Studies, 176
Centers for Disease Control, 29
Chelation (see EDTA)
Cheng, Tsung O., 360-361
Cheraskin, E., 31, 50, 100, 101, 120, 144, 203, 220, 240, 241, 262, 263, 264, 283, 304, 324-325, 389

Children
   of divorced parents questionnaire, 12
   stress questionnaire, 133-141
Cholesterol, 89-107
Cline, D. W., 390
Cognitive therapy, 203
Cognitive treatment, 191
Cohen, S. R., 180
Comprehensive Care Corporation, 76
Connor, S., 265
Cooper, Millie, 317, 326
Cooper, Kenneth H., 319, 326
Coronary heart disease (CHD), (see heart disease)
Cousins, Norman, 3, 67
   Anatomy of an Illness, 4, 67
Cox, N. H., 180
Creasey, W. A., 54
Crisp, A. H., 84
Crook, William G., 200, 205
Cypress, B. K., 32

D

Daniell, H. W., 284
Darlington, L. G., 67
Davis, W. H., 101
Department of Health and Human Services, 20
Depression, 188-193
   cognitive treatment, 191
   questionnaire, 190-191, 207
Diabetes mellitus, 14
Diamond, H., 390
Diet, 247-269, 350
   arthritis, 65, 67
   cancer, 43, 47, 51, 53, 54
   fatigue, 29, 34

questionnaires, 249-256, 265, 269
Disease
   diet, 51
Donoghue, S., 181
Duke, M. P., 11

E

Eating Attitudes Test (EAT), 77, 80, 84, 85
   questionnaire, 78-79
Eating Disorders Inventory (EDI), 80
Eckardt, M. J., 305
EDTA chelation
   arthritis, 70
   clinical change, 69
   emotional state, 206
   fatigue, 34
Ellis, F. R., 32
Emotional state, 206-207
Ennui, 24
Environment, 368
Environmental Protection Agency, 365
Epilogue, 371-372
Epsom District Hospital, 64
Eveningness questionnaire, 338-342, 346
Ewing, J. A., 305
Exercise (see physical activity)
Exhausted, 19
External health locus of control, 11, 14, 15
Eysenck, H. J., 285
Eysenck Personality Questionnaire, 285

F

Fabry, Paul, 261, 265
   folic acid, 48

FANTASTIC, 225-246
    questionnaire, 226-237, 245
Farquhar, John W., 194, 206, 323, 326
Fatigue, 19-39, 369
    adrenocortical, 36
    boredom, 37
    EDTA, 34
    hormones, 36
    iron deficiency, 30
    males, 30
    potassium, 35
    scale, 35
    women, 30
Faust, Volker, 361
Favazza, A. R., 306
Federal Bureau of Investigation, 375
Ferguson, T., 182
Fielding, J. E., 285
Financial health, 151-168
Fluids (see water)
Fonda, Jane, 75
Food and Drug Administration, 256
Freedman, Jonathan, 211
Freudenberger, Herbert J., 24-25, 33
Fries, James, 59, 68

G

Gabler, R., 366
Garfinkel, Paul E., 77, 85, 86
Garn, Stanley, 239, 241
Garner, David E., 77, 85, 86
German, D., 165
Ginter, E., 102
Goldberg, P., 344
Greenhalgh, R. M., 286

Greenwald, P., 55
Guilleminault, C., 345
Gutsy index, 10, 13

H

Hagan, R. D., 102
Hahn, Dale, B., 315, 327
Hales, D., 345
Hammond, C. E., 346
Hammond, E. S., 331
Happiness, 209-222
    questionnaire, 211, 213-216, 218, 220-221
Harper, Charles, 111
Harris, Seale, 110
Health
    financial, 151-168
    levels of, 376-379, 387
    locus of control
        definition, 4
    questionnaire, 380-383, 387
    workplace, 169-185
Heart disease, 193-198
    questionnaire, 195-197, 206
Hermann, W. J., Jr., 103
Herzog, D. B., 86
High density lipoprotein cholesterol (HDL), 92
Hochstim, J., 376
Hofeldt, F. D., 122
Hoffer, A., 68, 266
Holmes, Thomas, 144
Hormones,
    fatigue, 36
Horne, J. A., 337, 346
Horrobin, D. F., 306
Human Nutrition Information Service, 256

Human Synergistics, 176
Humphrey, J. H., 144
Hyperkinetics, 369
Hypoglycemia, 109-125
   questionnaire, 113

I

Iglehart, J. H., 182
Infection
   yeast, 200-202
Insomnia, 332-333
Internal health locus of control, 11, 14, 15

J

Jacobson, B., 87
Jaffe, Dennis T., 27-28, 33
Japanese Association of Industrial Health, 21
Jennings, C., 183
Jones, D. M., 367
Jordan-March, M., 11
Journal of the American Medical Association
   (JAMA), 65

K

Kals, W. S., 367
Kalter, N., 12
Kent, G. G., 13
Keys, Ralph, 10, 13
Knight, S., 165
Kohls, D. J., 104
Kolonel, L. N., 307
Kory, Robert, 376
Kozma, A., 220, 221

Kuntzleman, C. T., 327

L

Lacks, Patricia, 336, 347
Lancet, 64
Leveille, G., 266
Lifestyle questionnaire, 226-237, 240, 383-387, 388, 389
Light, 354, 369
    arthritis, 66-67
    cancer, 355
Locus of control, 3-16
    chance (CHLC), 9
    internal (IHLC), 9
    multidimensional (MHLC), 10
        internal, 11, 14, 15
        external, 11, 14, 15
    oral health, 13
    Powers (PHLC), 10
Loeb, M., 368
Loma Linda University, 301
Long, Ruth Yale, 257, 266
Low blood sugar (see hypoglycemia)
Low density lipoprotein cholesterol (LDL), 92

M

McDonagh, E. W., 34, 69, 104
McNelly, G. W., 21, 35
Machtey, I., 69
Marks, J., 267
Marlett, G. A., 287
MAST (Michigan Alcoholism Screening Test), 295-299, 306
Mattlin, E., 347

Medical examinations, 45
Medical News, 35, 287, 307
Medical World News, 181
Meier, Paul D., 190, 207
Memorial University of Newfoundland Scale of Happiness (MUNSH), 213-216, 220-221
Michigan Alcoholism Screening Test (MAST), 295-299, 306
Miles, Laughton, 345
Miller, G. Tyler, 356, 368
Miller, T. J., 166
Minirth, Frank B., 190, 207
Morgan, G. L., 288
Morningness questionnaire, 338-342, 346
MUNSH (Memorial University of Newfoundland Scale of Happiness), 213-216, 220-221

N

Narcolepsy, 333-334
National Anorexic Aid Society, Inc. (NAAS), 80
National Ambulatory Medical Care Survey (NAMCS), 32
National Association of Anorexia-Nervosa and Associated Disorders, Inc. (ANAD), 81
National Cancer Institute, 55
National Training Laboratory Institute (NTL), 177
Nature, 224, 238-239, 244, 261, 301
Newman, P. A., 87
Nicotinic acid
    arthritis, 68
Noise, 365-366, 367, 368
Non-smokers' Rights Association, 174
Novaco, R. W., 145
Null, G., 308
Nurture, 224, 238-239, 244, 261, 301

Nutrition, 34

O

Odetti, P., 105
Office on Smoking and Health, 283, 289
Oral health, 13
Orthodontics
    questionnaire, 11
Ostberg, Olov, 337
Osteoarthritis (OA), 58
Ott, John Nash, 355, 369
Owl/lark questionnaire, 338-342

P

Paffenbarger, R. S., 391
Paine, W. S., 36
Palmore, E., 391
Pauling, Linus, 49
Payne, Wayne A., 315, 327
Pelletier, K. R., 184
Perez, Carla, 160
Pesznecker, B. L., 145
Pfeiffer, C. C., 267
Phillipson, B. E., 105
Phoenix House, 176
Photobiology, 355
Physical activity, 45, 313-330
    arthritis, 66-67
    questionnaires 314-316, 317-318, 323
Pleas, J., 328
Poleliakhoff, A., 36
Ponderal index, 53
Porter, S., 166
Potassium, 35

Powers, J. S., 308
Powers, P. S., 88
Pratt, L., 392
Prentice, W. E., 328
President's Council on Physical Fitness and Sports, 175
Prevention
   primary, 46
      of occurence, 46
      or recurrence, 46
   secondary, 47
Prevention Magazine, 268, 380
Preventive dentistry
   questionnaire, 13
Primary prevention, 46
Problems, 17-18
Prologue, 1
Psychodietetics, 122, 144, 192, 205, 220, 304
Psychological Assessment Resources, 80

Q

Questionnaires
   alcoholism, 302
      CAGE, 295, 305-306
      MAST, 295-299, 306, 308
      teenager, 302
   Alpha test, 257, 268
   American Banker's Association, 153, 165
   American Medical Association, 130-132
   anger, 145
   Angers Happiness, 219
   anorexia nervosa, 78-79, 84
   arthritis, 59, 60, 61
   Beck Depression Inventory (BDI), 202, 203
   bulemia, 78-79

burnout, 26-27, 33, 37, 38
CAGE, 294-295, 305-306
cancer, 43, 48, 54
carbohydrates, 258-260, 269
Center for Science in the Public Interest, 249-256
children of divorced parents, 12
children's stress, 133-141
depression, 190-191, 203, 207
diet, 249-256, 265, 269
EAT (Eating Attitudes Test), 78-79, 84, 85
emotional, 257, 268
emotional state, 206-207
eveningness, 338-342, 346
Eysenck Personality, 285
FANTASTIC, 226-237, 244, 245
fatigue, 21-24, 31, 39
financial, 153, 165
Food Fix, 257, 269
good and bad cholesterol, 93-95, 107
Hamilton Rating Scale for Depression, 193
happiness, 213-216, 218-219, 220, 221
health, 376-379, 380-383, 387
heart disease, 195-197, 206
hypoglycemia, 113
insomnia, 332-333
lark, 338-342
leisurely stroll, 328
levels of health, 376-379, 387
lifestyle, 226-237, 240, 383-387, 388, 389
locus of control, 6, 15, 16
MAST (Michigan Alcoholism Screening Test), 295-299, 306, 308
mental, 257, 268
Michigan Alcoholism Screening Test (MAST), 295-299, 306, 308

morningness, 338-342, 246
MUNSH (Memorial University of Newfoundland Scale of Happiness), 213-216, 220-221
narcoleptic, 333-334
orthodontic, 5, 11
owl, 338-342
PAR-Q, 329
preventive dentistry, 13
physical activity, 315-318, 323, 326, 327, 328
radiation, 357-358, 369
restless leg syndrome, 334-335
shopaholic, 160
sleep, 332-337, 345, 348
sleep hygiene, 336
stress, 130-132, 144
sugar intake, 258-260, 269
teenage
    alcoholism, 302
    FANTASTIC, 231-234
    tobacco, 279-282, 289
tiredness, 35
tobacco, 274-278, 285, 289
Total Life Stress Test (TLS), 243
vanity, 317-318, 326
walking, 323, 326, 327, 328
weather, 362-363, 367, 370
workplace, 172, 174, 182
yeast infection, 200-201, 205-206

R

Radiation, 356, 369
    high level, 356
    low level, 356
    questionnaire, 357-358
Rahe, Richard H., 144, 146, 147

Raudsepp, Eugene, 133
Ray, M. B., 14
Regestein, Q. R., 347
Register, U. D., 309
Restless leg syndrome, 334-335
Reuler, J. B., 70
Rheumatoid arthritis (RA), 58
Riordan, H. D., 123
Rippon, J. W., 207
Roberts, H. J., 112, 124
Roberts, Sam E., 112
Rosen, S., 370
Rotert, Monique, 336
Ruggiero, R., 124
Ruhenstroth-Bauer, G., 361
Russeck, H., 147

S

Sandler, D. P., 290
Schauss, Alexander G., 112
Schlenk, E. A., 14
Schoenthaler, Stephen J., 112
Scott, Cynthia, 27-28, 33
Scurvy, 70
Secondary prevention, 47
Section A: the Prologue, 1
Section B: the Problems, 17
Section C: the Solutions, 223
Section D: the Epilogue, 371
Selye, H., 148
Serum cholesterol
   arginine, 104
   EDTA, 104
   lysine, 104
   magnesium, 101

    niacin, 105
    normal range, 91
    sitting, 98, 103
    standing, 98, 103
    tryptophan, 104
    vitamin C, 102
    vitamin E, 103
Service, J. F., 125
Shaver, Philip, 211, 222
Shealy, C. N., 243
Sherk, C., 244
Simonton, C. O., 55
Sleep, 44, 331-348
Sloan, L., 167
Smart vitamins, 102
Smoking, 29, 43, 271-291
    questionnaires, 274-278, 279-282, 285, 289
Solutions, Section C
Spondylitis, ankylosing, 3
Stamler, R., 184
Stewart, G. T., 200, 329
Stokes, B., 393
Stoltz, Sandra Gordon, 257, 269
Stone, I., 393
Stress, 28, 44, 127-149
    job, 36
    questionnaire, 130-132, 144
Stress Test, 243
Strickland, B. R., 14
Stuman, F. A., 329
Surgeon-General's Report, 226, 277, 286, 290

T

Tache, J., 148
teenager

alcohol questionnaire, 302
FANTASTIC, 231-234
smoking questionnaire, 279-282, 289
Tired, 19
Tired blood, 31
Tiredness
vitamin B_{12}, 33
questionnaire, 35
Tobacco, 47, 271-291
questionnaire, 274-278
teenage questionnaire, 279-282, 289
Tocopherol
arthritis, 69
Total Life Stress Test (TLS), 243
Tran, Z. V., 106
Triglycerides, 90
Trowell, H. 269
Truss, C. O., 208
Tumors (see cancer)

U

Ultraviolet (UV), 354
University of Alabama at Birmingham Multipurpose Arthritis Center, 64
University of California at Los Angeles, 75

V

Vigderman, P., 37
Vitamin B_{12}
tiredness, 33
Vitamin C, 393
arthritis, 70, 71
cancer, 49, 54
fatigue, 31

Vitamin C Connection, 31, 54
Vitamins
   smart, 102
Vogan, H., Jayne, 171

W

Wallston, Barbara Strudler, 10, 15, 16
Wallston, Kenneth A., 10, 15, 16
Warter, P. J., 70
Washington Business Group on Health, 29
Water, 224, 225, 351-353, 366
   arthritis, 67
Weary, 19
Weather, 360, 364, 367
   questionnaire, 362-363, 367, 370
Weight, 43, 52, 73-88
Welch, I. D., 38
Williams, R. J., 310
Williams, R. R., 244
Wilson, Douglas M.C., 226, 245
Wood, P. D., 93, 106
Wood, V., 222
Workplace
   health, 169-185
Worksite Health Promotion, 177
Worn out, 19

Y

Yanker, G. D., 329
Yeast infection, 200-202, 205, 208
Yoshitake, H., 21, 38

Z

Zajonc, R. B., 245

ABOUT THE PUBLISHER

Bio-Communications Press is a service of The Olive W. Garvey Center for the Improvement of Human Functioning, Inc. The Center is a non-profit medical, research and educational organization funded through grants from corporations and foundations and contributions from individuals.

The Center has established three major divisions to carry out its mission of seeking to help stimulate an epidemic of health. These are the ABNA Clinical Research Center, The Bio-Communications Research Institute and The Bio-Medical Synergistics Education Institute.

To learn more about The Center, pictured below, just send your note of request together with a stamped self-addressed #10 envelope to:

The Center
3100 N. Hillside Avenue
Wichita, Kansas 67219 USA

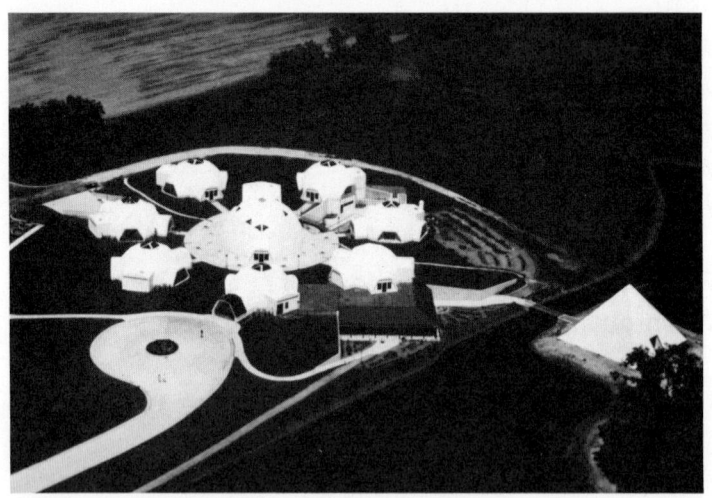

The 21st Century Center Master Facility of 8 geodesic domes and pyramid

Bio-Communications Press

THERE'S MORE

Bio-Communications Press fulfills a unique niche by publishing fascinating books for select audiences. These books are written by skilled professionals who have demonstrated both a profound interest in their subject matter and the capacity to clearly communicate that interest in an understandable way.

Although our books are not for everyone, we believe what we publish makes a valuable addition to the personal library of anyone who appreciates being well informed on the subject matter they contain.

Our current list of published books:

Medical Mavericks, Volume One–Hugh Riordan, M.D.
The Schizophrenias: Ours to Conquer–Carl Pfeiffer, Ph.D., M.D.
The Vitamin C Controversy: Questions and Answers–Emanuel Cheraskin, M.D., D.M.D.
The Wonderful World Within You–Roger Williams, Ph.D.

Soon to be released:

Electrodynamic Man–Leonard Ravitz, M.D.
Hypnosis, Acupuncture & Pain–Maurice Tinterow, M.D., Ph.D.
Medical Mavericks, Volume Two–Hugh Riordan, M.D.

To receive a list of books currently available from Bio-Communications Press or to be among the first to know when a new book is about to be released, just return the coupon today.

Bio-Communications Press, 3100 N. Hillside,
Wichita, Kansas 67219 U.S.A.

Please send me information about available books.

NAME _____

ADDRESS _____

CITY _____

STATE _____ ZIP CODE _____